Luciana Ribeiro Campos

Taxation of Water Charging

Luciana Ribeiro Campos

Taxation of Water Charging

Environmental taxation as an instrument for preserving water resources

ScienciaScripts

Imprint

Any brand names and product names mentioned in this book are subject to trademark, brand or patent protection and are trademarks or registered trademarks of their respective holders. The use of brand names, product names, common names, trade names, product descriptions etc. even without a particular marking in this work is in no way to be construed to mean that such names may be regarded as unrestricted in respect of trademark and brand protection legislation and could thus be used by anyone.

Cover image: www.ingimage.com

This book is a translation from the original published under ISBN 978-613-9-68198-3.

Publisher:
Sciencia Scripts
is a trademark of
Dodo Books Indian Ocean Ltd. and OmniScriptum S.R.L publishing group

120 High Road, East Finchley, London, N2 9ED, United Kingdom
Str. Armeneasca 28/1, office 1, Chisinau MD-2012, Republic of Moldova, Europe
Printed at: see last page
ISBN: 978-620-7-72352-2

To Fabio, my inspiration in everything I do. My love, you bring light and truth, you dedicate love to me and keep me from uncertainty, you accompany me with serenity, dedication and patience... without you I would be nothing.... because "even if I spoke in the tongues of men and of angels, and had not love, I should be as sounding brass, or as a tinkling bell" (Co 13:1). I love you.

To our children Rafael and Mariana, who are the most perfect expression of this love honored and blessed by God.

SUMMARY

Introduce.

Freshwater is increasingly taking center stage in scientific studies. This is because humanity's current lifestyle is incompatible with maintaining the quality and quantity of water resources. A change in the way these resources are managed, making the various uses compatible with their preservation and conservation, is the way forward.

With this conservationist aim in mind, Law 9.433/97 inaugurated a new way of managing water resources. The first step taken by the law was the recognition that water is an exhaustible good, with economic value, which serves various uses - which must be made compatible and prioritized if there is a situation of scarcity - which overcomes the mentality that it is inexhaustible, that is, a renewable source and therefore not economically valuable.

The second step was to establish a form of participatory and decentralized management, taking into account the unity of water bodies. Participatory management helps to establish the environmental good (water) as a diffuse good, which therefore requires the direct intervention of all its holders, to the extent that the government and the community are jointly responsible for the preservation of environmental goods. Decentralized management brings government action closer to the local level of problems, enabling immediate action. This form of action is coordinated by a centralized and uniform policy, taking into account the unity of the hydrographic basin and the shared hydro-environmental impacts.

In line with the participatory and decentralized way of managing water resources, guided by a centralized policy drawn up by the Union, which considers the unity of the environmental asset, Law 9.433/97 structures a national water resources system, creating bodies and instituting instruments through which this national policy will be achieved.

Among the instruments devised by the legislator was the charge for the permitted use of water resources, or simply the water charge, which aims to control the quantity and quality of water resources in order to preserve them for present and future generations.

From the outset, it should be made clear that this new way of charging for water is not to be confused with the charges levied by sanitation companies in the states and municipalities, which supply urban centers with treated water. This is not the case regulated by Law 9.433/97. Charges are levied for water collected for treatment, i.e. what the sanitation company itself collects for treatment purposes (raw water), which is just one of the many possible uses for water resources.

Other uses are also charged, such as water abstraction for industrial uses, irrigation uses, agribusiness uses or the emission of effluents from industrial waste, sanitation, ballast water disposal (art. 2, XVII, Law 9.966/2000), among others.

It can be seen, then, that the water charges that Law 9.433/97 established cannot be confused with the charges levied for the water treatment service, since the legislator's intention in creating this and the other instruments is to implement the National Policy aimed at ensuring that current and future generations have the necessary availability of water, at quality standards appropriate to their respective uses; the possibility of the rational and integrated use of water resources, including waterway transport, with a view to sustainable development; and the search for prevention and defense against critical hydrological events of natural origin or resulting from the inappropriate use of natural resources (art. 2° of Law 9.433/97).[1]

The intention, as stated in the legislation itself, is not to pay for a public water supply service, but to encourage a culture of preservation in the various sectors of society, so that, even in the face of multiple uses, the quantity and quality of water resources are preserved in perpetuity.

With the realization that the aim of the law was to lead users to act consciously in

---

[1] Law 13.501 of 2017 added a fourth objective to the National Water Resources Policy: "IV - to encourage and promote the capture, preservation and use of rainwater".

relation to water resources, and not to charge for a "service" or for the use of a good, we can see another nuance of the institute itself, created with the law, which is the difficulty of establishing its legal nature.

A critical look at the figure created by Law 9.433/97 raises countless questions about the nature of the new institute. The first question arises when it is observed that we are, in principle, dealing with a "public good" (we use quotation marks to denote that we do not fully agree with this classification of goods into public and private whenever we are talking about environmental goods, which we consider to be diffuse goods, we prefer the designation environmental goods or diffuse goods, which we will now use) and the use of "public good" is, as a rule, associated with public employment[2] .

A more detailed analysis will show that charging for water, according to Law 9.433/97, does not behave like this, because it is not only established by law ("ex lege" obligation), but also has an intrinsic purpose to be achieved, which is even reflected in the linking of the funds collected to the achievement of this purpose (conserving water resources for present and future generations).

In addition, the law protects the existential minimum, insofar as it exempts from licensing and, consequently, exempts from charging the uses intended to satisfy the needs of small populations, distributed in rural areas; the derivations, abstractions and releases considered insignificant; the accumulations of volumes of water considered insignificant (insignificant consumption compatible with the uses intended to guarantee survival and human dignity). The immunity of the minimum existential does not exist in the field of public

---

[2] We consider the synonymy between tariffs and public charges (ATALIBA, Geraldo. Hipotese de Incidencia Tributaria. 6 ed., 3ª tiragem, Sao Paulo: Malheiros, 2002, p. 145; MEIRELES, Hely Lopes. Brazilian Administrative Law. 14. ed., Sao Paulo: Malheiros Editores, 1989, p. 346; DI PIETRO, Maria Sylvia Zanella. Administrative Law. 16. ed., Sao Paulo: Atlas, 2003, p. 244; AMARO, Luciano. Brazilian Tax Law. 9. ed., Sao Paulo: Saraiva, 2003. p. 43), despite recognizing that there are authors who consider tariffs to be a generic term (VERLI, Fabiano. Fees and public charges. Sao Paulo: Editora Revista dos Tribunais, 2005, p. 41) or tariff as an autonomous institute (MELO, Celso Antonio Bandeira de. Course in Administrative Law. 13. ed., rev., ampl. e atual., Sao Paulo: Malheiros Editores, 2001, p. 690).

employment. All of these characteristics distance the present figure from the one designated by the doctrine as prego publico.

The translation of the 1934 Water Code can also lead to misunderstandings and make the interpretation of Law 9.433/97 more difficult. In fact, the legislation in force until the advent of the latter law treated water as an inexhaustible public good, the economic value of which was directly related to private property or hydro-energy potential. As a result, the Water Code (art. 36, § 2) allowed the use of a public asset to be remunerated through the establishment of a public charge, with no specific purpose other than to supply the public coffers with funds.

Therefore, the doctrinal landscape is not easy to establish without further study the legal nature of the water charge established in Law 9.433/97 as a public charge or as a tax. The importance of establishing the legal nature lies in the consequences of each of the regimes to which each of these species is subject.

The tax legal system is bound by strict legality, anteriority, non-retroactivity and the prohibition of the confiscation effect, among other principles and rules. Public procurement, on the other hand, is subject to market logic, to the principle of supply and demand, and is established, as a rule, by the will of the parties.

On the other hand, it has to be considered that water, as an essential commodity for life, should not be tied to a market policy that does not protect and enable access even for those who cannot afford it. It is worth remembering the incompatibility of the public service system with charging for water, drawing a parallel with the provision of public services by electricity companies. There is a considerable amount of doctrine and jurisprudence that admits cutting off the supply of electricity in the face of the user's breach of contract. Using this reasoning by analogy, it would be possible to cancel the grant for abstraction, derivation, extraction or emission in the event of default, which would be absurd in cases where it is essential to protect the ecological minimum (not just the existential minimum or vital minimum).

The study of water charges is the purpose of this dissertation, in the light not only of Environmental Law, but also of Tax Law, in an interdisciplinary and transdisciplinary analysis of the subject[3] .

In an attempt to investigate the legal nature of this institute, we realized that tax law is a great ally of the environment and specifically of water resources. Today, it is no longer possible to ignore the environmental crisis, which is the result of predatory practices and the prevailing atd thinking. This view gave rise to the notion that all environmental resources were inexhaustible and thus exploited, until the international community cried out in 1972 at the Stockholm Conference.

From that moment to today, thinking has evolved towards the gradual recognition of the fragility of the great ecosystem called Earth, but on the other hand, environmental degradation has also evolved. On the international and national scene, significant efforts have been made to contain it, including the Kyoto Protocol and the Biodiversity Convention.

In order to achieve the above objective, the work has been structured into seven chapters. The first chapter looks at the many uses of water and its importance to society, and provides some statistical data to demonstrate the water crisis. Then, in the second chapter, an effort is made to provide a historicized view of water in the national and international legal order.

The third chapter presents some data on the management models found in continental Europe, in particular identifying the legal nature of charging in French, German and Spanish law.

In chapter four, we propose a rereading of constitutional competencies in water

---

[3] NICOLESCU, Barsarab. Transdisciplinary evolution: the university condition for sustainable development. Available at: http://perso.club-internet.fr/nicol/ciret/bulletin/b 12c8por.htm. Accessed on August 1, 2005.

matters, laying the initial foundations for recognizing the tax nature of the levy established in Law 9.433/97. The next step is a general analysis of the system of water resources envisioned in the Law, and other legal foundations that corroborate the tax nature of the levy are listed in the fifth chapter.

The sixth chapter explores the economic, ethical and legal foundations that allow us to affirm that environmental taxation, especially in its extra-fiscal nature, is the best way to protect the environment and water resources. The problem of tax immunities is addressed in the light of the theory of the existential minimum and the ecological minimum, in the context of environmental taxation. It is found that water resources intended for human consumption and animal watering are protected by this immunity clause.

The зёйшо chapter presents an analysis of charging in the light of tax law theory. This chapter discusses the elements of the definition of a tax that allow us to characterize the levy in the Water Law as a tax. It then identifies the most appropriate type of tax to deal with the peculiarities of the charge in the Water Law. It is noted that the contribution for intervention in the economic domain fits the hypothesis of incidence provided for in Law 9.433/97. Finally, the hypothesis of levy is broken down in order to legally recognize its various aspects.

Chapter 1

Water: importance and uses.

Water, a colorless, odorless and insipid liquid, is essential to life, because without it there is no respiration, reproduction, photosynthesis, chemosynthesis, *habitats* and ecological niches for the majority of existing species[4] .

Most countries went from the point where water resources were considered unlimited to the point where they had to be used with caution and protected from pollution[5] .

It should be noted that the culture of free water, well portrayed by the Roman playwright, Titus Muccius Plautus, for whom "the day, the water, the sun, the moon, the night - these are things I don't have to buy with money", demonstrates that quantitative limitations and pollution were not factors considered by many civilizations[6] . So, when people needed water, they went to the nearest water source to get it[7] .

In ancient history, up until 440 years after the founding of Rome, the demand for water was satisfied by tapping the River Tiber through ponds and fountains. The growth of the Roman city led to the construction of the first water supply system in history (312 B.C.), so that water reached the population through aqueducts instead of being collected from[8] . Julius Frontanius, as Rome's Commissar of Water (97 AD), managed a complex system of Roman

---

[4] FIORILLO, Celso Antonio Pacheco; and RODRIGUES, Marcelo Abelha. Manual of Environmental Law and Applicable Legislation. 2. ed. Sao Paulo: MaxLimonad, 1999, p. 286.

[5] CAPONERA, Dante A. Principles of water law and administration: national and international. Rotterdam: Balkema, 1992, p. 2.

[6] CAMPOS, Nilson; STUDART, Ticiana. Charging for water use. *In:* Gestao de aguas: principios e praticas. Nilson Campos e Ticiana Studart (orgs.), 2. ed. Porto Alegre: ABRH, 2003, p. 113.

[7] Ibid., p. 113.

[8] CAMPOS, Nilson; STUDART, Ticiana. A cobranga ..., p. 113.

aqueducts that collected water from remote sources and led it to reservoirs distributed throughout the city, and his work *De aquedutuë* is a reference point for many management systems even today .[9]

The Middle Ages brought a culture of a certain dread of water and, consequently, less demand for it. "Hygiene habits, such as bathing, were not practiced with the frequency recommended today"[10] . There were no great advances in water management during this period.

With the Industrial Revolution, the concentration of the population in cities began to generate serious problems in terms of water quality, a problem that is only getting worse today. The lack of sewage systems in these centers, as they are today, reduces the quality of the water and leads to ever higher costs for its treatment[11] .

It is estimated that, in order to guarantee a reasonable quality of life, approximately eighty liters of water would be needed per inhabitant, considering the various uses, including domestic[12] .

Of the world's fresh water, 73% is used in agriculture, 21% in industry and 6% as drinking water. The water used in agriculture is wasted enormously, as 60% of it is lost before it even reaches the plant[13] . Irrigation is the use that consumes the most water and, if it is used intensively, it can lead to serious conflicts, not only those involving irrigation but also those relating to other uses (e.g. public supply), leading to serious disputes. Indeed, domestic consumption alone has grown more than 35 times in the last three decades and has quadrupled since 1940[14] . An inevitable conflict between the various uses is looming, but it can be avoided

---

[9] CAMPOS, Nilson. Water Management: new visions and paradigms. *In:* Water management: principles and practices. Nilson Campos and Ticiana Studart (eds.), 2. ed. Porto Alegre: ABRH, 2003, p. 21.
[10] Ibid., p. 22.
[11] Ibid., p. 22.
[12] SOUZA, Luciana Cordeiro. Waters and their protection. Curitiba: Jurua, 2004, p. 117.
[13] ANTUNES, Paulo de Bessa. Environmental Law. Editora Lumen Juris: Rio de Janeiro, 2006, p. 687.
[14] CAMPOS, Nilson. Management ... p. 113.

if more efficient irrigation techniques are adopted in terms of water use. In short, there is an urgent need for the rational use of water.

Since 1900, the amount of freshwater used has multiplied sixfold, while the population has doubled. Agriculture is by far the biggest consumer of fresh water, mainly due to the development of irrigation. It currently accounts for around two-thirds of total consumption - a proportion that is only expected to decline very slightly from 2025 onwards. Therefore, any reduction in consumption requires an improvement in irrigation techniques[15].

If this trend doesn't change, the amount of freshwater available *per capita per* year will fall from the current 6,800m3 to 4,800m3 in 2025. This calculation is based on a fairly theoretical global volume of disposable water: all the water that flows into rivers, minus the effects of evaporation and infiltration. It therefore ignores the minimum quantities of water needed to keep aquatic ecosystems alive, water that is difficult to access and, above all, the consequences of the unequal distribution of this resource on the planet[16].

The level of 1,700m3 of water available *per capita per* year is the limit of "water stress", above which there can be frequent shortages. Below the scarcity line, set at 1,000m3 *per capita per year,* serious problems arise in the areas of production and agriculture, among others. If nothing is done, the number of people suffering from water stress will rise from 2.3 to 3.5 billion by 2025, when 2.4 billion people will suffer from scarcity. Today, the latest figure is 1.7 billion[17].

Given this situation, it must be considered that any use of water must be planned and managed, otherwise there will be harmful side effects on the water itself or on other natural resources. Dante A. Caponera believes that the development and conservation of water

---

[15] UNESCO. Great rivers: from conflict to sharing. Infographics: a growing scarcity. *In:* O Correio Unesco. n° 12, ano 29, Rio de Janeiro: FGV Editora, December, 2001, p. 20.
[16] Ibid., p. 20.
[17] Ibid., p. 20.

resources depends to a large extent on the effectiveness of water laws[18] . This is because the growing demand for water, as opposed to the growing reduction in its quantity to meet demand, puts pressure on the social system to develop efficient legal mechanisms capable of reallocating available water from less productive uses to more desirable uses for society[19] . Indeed, studies show that this resource will become considerably scarcer in the coming decades and that developing countries will be the first to be affected. The more demand increases, the more water becomes a source of conflict among consumers. Thousands of people are already suffering the effects of its lack and, unless we completely change the way we view and manage this resource, the damage will be enormous, both for the planet and its inhabitants.

In view of the statistics on the scarcity of this natural resource and taking into account its economic indispensability, it is necessary to place it in a sustainable context, i.e. the use of water must be rational, in order to guarantee it for present and future generations, imposing on the Government the duty to use all available instruments to achieve this end, especially environmental taxation.

---

[18] "Since the negative effects can be avoided through the enactment of adequate water legislation and the establishment of an appropriate water administration, it may be said that the success of development and conservation of water resources in any country depends to a large extent on the effectiveness of its water laws". (CAPONERA, Dante A. Principles of water law and administration: national and international. Rotterdam: Balkema, 1992, p.2).

[19] "Water demands for drinking purposes grow in parallel with population growth, while modern standards of living require increased amounts of water for domestic uses such as gardening and recreational purposes. Likewise, the increasing world population necessitates more water for irrigation and livestock in order to satisfy increasing food requirements." (Ibid., p.1).

Chapter 2

Historical aspects of water policies.

2.1 International scenario. 2.2. National scenario.

2.1. International scenario.

By historically situating the process of building the right to access water and the form of management, it will be possible to better understand the figure of charging.

Christian Caubet informs us that the historical milestone of the discussion on water was the year 1815, when the Congress of Vienna established the parameters of European relations and served to consolidate several statutes of the utmost importance, "restoration of the system of the five great European powers; establishment of the statute of diplomatic representatives; proclamation of the illicit trade in blacks; establishment of freedom of navigation on the 'international' European river waters - Danube, Meuse, Moselle, Neckar and Rhine"[20] . Thus, the first discussion on water was motivated by navigation on river waters and not the preservation of their quality and quantity, so that the use in evidence was transportation.

It was at the end of the 19th century that another major use for water resources emerged, namely the production of electricity[21] . "At first, the construction of dams, which could prevent the use of boats, was carried out in places where it was not an obstacle: in mountainous areas, upstream of the place where navigation becomes naturally possible"[22] .

---

[20] CAUBET, Christian G. Freshwater in international relations. Barueri: Manole, 2006, p. XX.
[21] CAUBET, ChristianG. Aagua ....Ibid., p. XX.
[22] Ibid., p. XX.

This use did not conflict with navigation; the culture of open water was maintained.

In fact, the debate in the international community about water and the need to conserve it only took place in 1949 at the United Nations Scientific Conference on the Conservation and Use of Natural Resources, whose central themes were the degradation of oceans, rivers and seas, industrial pollution, the management of hazardous waste, rural migration to urban centers, climate change and nuclear development.

In 1964, the United Nations Conference on Trade and Development (UNCTAD) discussed the use of maritime waters from the perspective of their economic exploitation. An exclusively preservationist approach to natural resources was set aside in order to emphasize the economic use of maritime waters. From UNCTAD onwards, it became clear that environmental concerns were widespread across the planet.

In 1965, UNESCO declared the International Hydrological Decade. This was a scientific program with the aim of carrying out an assessment of the world's water resources and promoting their rational use[23] .

In 1971, the UN Economic Commission for Europe held a Symposium on Environmental Problems in Prague, Czechoslovakia. In this document, for the first time, there was talk of punishing polluters.

In Stockholm, Sweden, the United Nations Conference on the Human Environment was held in 1972[24] . This conference consolidated the foundations of the modern environmental policy adopted by all countries, with greater or lesser rigor, in their particular legislations. This conference led to the preparation of a study on the environmental situation in the world: the Brundtland Report, also known as "Our Common Future", was published in April 1987 and its recommendations were adopted in more than 100 countries, according to the

---

[23] CUNHA, Luis Veiga da. Half a century of perceptions of water in international politics. *In:* SOROMENHO-MARQUES, Viriato. The Challenge of Water in the 21st Century: Between Conflict and Cooperation. Lisbon: Noticia Editorial: 2003, p. 34.
[24] MUKAI, Toshio. Systematized environmental law. Rio de Janeiro: Forense Universitaria, 2005, p. 181.

reality of each nation.

With regard to water specifically, the Stockholm Declaration only expressly referred to it in one of its 26 principles, although many of these contained implicit references to it as an environmental element[25] .

In 1973, a Conference on the Law of the Sea began. But it wasn't until December 1982, in Montego Bay, Jamaica, that the Conference put the United Nations Convention on the Law of the Sea up for signature. Brazil ratified the Convention in December 1988.

Following the results of the Law of the Sea Conference, the UN convened the first United Nations Water Conference, which was held in March 1977 in Mar del Plata, Argentina. This was the first specialized meeting to deal with water problems. At this meeting, the emergence of a long-term water crisis was indicated, which could only be alleviated through the adoption of integrated water management programs[26] .

The main aim of the Mar del Plata conference was to get the necessary measures adopted at local, regional, national and international level to avoid global water crises by the end of the century, so that the world can have good quality quantities of this resource, adequate to meet the needs of a growing population that aspires to better economic and social conditions for all[27] . The Mar del Plata Action Plan was then drawn up. From this plan emerged the International Drinking Water Supply and Sanitation Decade. The UN Conference on Human Settlements - HABITAT, held in 1976 in Vancouver, Canada, also approved the recommendation, which stated that all countries should make efforts to provide drinking water and adequate sanitation services universally by 1990.

The International Drinking Water and Sanitation Decade was proclaimed by the UN in November 1980, with the aim of improving and promoting the coverage of drinking water and

---

[25] CUNHA, Luis Veiga da. Meio seculo..., p. 35.
[26] MACHADO, Paulo Affonso Leme. Water Resources - Brazilian and International Law. Sao Paulo: Malheiros Ediotres, 2002, p. 131.
[27] CUNHA, Luis Veiga da. op. cit., p. 36.

basic sanitation services for as many people as possible, especially those sectors located in the

suburbs of cities or in rural areas.

In 1983, an important step was taken in the defense of the environment, with the

creation of the World Commission on Environment and Development within the UN. Its aim,

in general terms, was to re-examine the environmental issue by interrelating it with the issue of

development and, in addition, to propose a global action program.

In New Эё1ЬI, India, in 1990, the conclusions of the Decade of Water activities were

presented. It was noted that the expected results had not been achieved. However, some

positive points can be highlighted: professionals in the sanitary engineering sector improved

their knowledge and certain endemic waterborne diseases were minimized or eradicated.

The UN held the second major International Conference on Water and the Environment

in Dublin, Ireland, in January 1992. It was considered that the situation of water resources was

moving quite dramatically towards a critical point. At this conference, it was stated that the

optimization of water resources can only be achieved through political commitment and the

participation of civil society. As a result of the Dublin Conference, recommendations and an

action program were produced under the title "Water and Sustainable Development". The

Declaration produced in Dublin states in four principles that:

> 1. Freshwater is a finite and vulnerable resource that is essential for ensuring life, development and the environment.
> 2. Water development and management must be based on a participatory approach at all levels, involving users, planners and political decision-makers.
> 3. Women play a central role in the supply, management and protection of water.
> 4. Water has an economic value in its various competitive uses and should be recognized as an economic good[28].

Dublin also highlighted the relationship between water and the alleviation of poverty

and disease; the protection of and measures against natural disasters; the conservation and

---

[28] CUNHA, Luis Veiga da. Meio sĕculo..., p. 37.

reuse of water; sustainable urban development; agricultural production and the supply of drinking water to rural areas; the protection of aquatic systems and cross-border issues and recognized the existence of geopolitical conflicts over the ownership of water basins.

In 1992, the United Nations Conference on Environment and Development was held in Rio de Janeiro, Brazil[29] . This conference recognized a situation in which environmental concerns came to occupy a central position on the national political agenda. The strategic document produced at this conference is Agenda 21, which, unlike the Stockholm Conference, devotes an entire chapter to water (Chapter 18). It recognizes that the widespread scarcity, gradual destruction and worsening pollution of water resources in many regions of the world, together with the progressive implementation of incompatible activities, require integrated planning and management of these resources. This integration must cover all types of interrelated bodies of freshwater, including both surface and groundwater, and take due account of both quantitative and qualitative aspects. However, the focus on water resources was predominantly centered on the issues of pollution and biodiversity, which is somewhat insufficient for an efficient water management policy. In this document, the concept of sustainable development is extended to water. Chapter 18 proposes a line of programs and strategies to be adopted in relation to water:

The following program areas are proposed for the freshwater sector:
a) Development and integrated management of water resources;
b) Assessment of water resources;
c) Protection of water resources, water quality and aquatic ecosystems;
d) Drinking water supply and sanitation;
e) Water and sustainable urban development;
f) Water for sustainable food production and sustainable rural development;

---

[29] ZUMBROICH, Thomas. The European Union's Basic Water Directive as a Result of Changing Awareness in the Protection of Water Resources. *In:* Local Agenda 21 - participatory management of water resources. Angela Kuster, Klaus Hermanns (org.), Fortaleza: Konrad Adenauer Foundation, 2006, p. 25.

Another event worth highlighting in this historical journey is the World Water Forum, which is held every three years. This international meeting was founded in 1996, within the framework of the World Water Council, to discuss the main issues related to water management. The 1st Forum was held in 1997 in Marrakech, Morocco; the 2nd Forum in The Hague, Holland, in 2000 and the 3rd World Water Forum was held concurrently in Kyoto, Shiga and Osaka, Japan, in 2003. The IV Forum was held in Mexico.

ªThe Forum discusses the actions taken by different countries to implement the integrated management of water resources and seeks solutions that will enable the international community to achieve the objectives of the Millennium Declaration, held in September 2000 in New York during the 55th Session of the United Nations, and those of the World Summit on Sustainable Development, held in Johannesburg in September 2002, which aim to halve the number of people without access to drinking water and basic sanitation by 2015.

In Kyoto, an Internet debate mechanism called the Water Media Network was created.

The UN General Assembly Resolution of December 20, 2000 declared 2003 to be the International Year of Freshwater. The aim was to raise public awareness of the importance of using and managing water resources.

To conclude this section, it is important to note that, especially since the 1990s, major international events have been held, as seen above, in which water has once again become a priority issue. In fact, it has been said that "20 years after the Mar del Plata Conference, there has not been another conference dedicated to the issue of water, which is an indication that it

---

[30] United Nations Conference on Environment and Development. 3. ed., Brasilia: Senado Federal, Subsecretaria de Edigoes Tecnicas, 2001.

has, in a way, ceased to be a priority issue".[31] Since Dublin, water has been considered a strategic asset, which is reflected in Brazilian legislation. There is a worldwide realization that these are finite resources, even though the perpetuation of life on earth depends on them infinitely. A paradigm shift is beginning to take place.

2.2. National scene.

The Afonsinas Ordinances and the Manoelinas Ordinances do not deal specifically with water. The former deals with environmental issues only in passing and the latter has a slightly more detailed protectionist approach, in that it introduces "the concept of environmental zoning - prohibiting the hunting of partridges, hares and rabbits in certain places - and there was the addition of notions of the theory of reparation of ecological damage in an advanced manner - stipulating the *quantum of* compensation according to the value of the tree".[32]

Thus, the first legal framework for water resources is the Philippine Ordinances of 1580, when Portugal was under Spanish rule. These legal texts showed concern about the scarcity of water, a situation that characterized the peninsula. They provided for very severe penalties for those who polluted or used water resources without proper authorization[33] . This

---

[31] CUNHA, Luis Veiga da. Meio seculo..., p. 38.

[32] ALMEIDA, Caroline Correa de. Historical evolution of the legal protection of water in Brazil. Jus Navigandi, Tersina, a. 7, n. 60, nov. 2002. Available at: http://jus2.uol.com.br/doutrina/texto.asp?id=3421. Accessed on: March 3, 2006.

[33] Ordenagoes Filipinas: Book 5, Title LXXXVIII: S. - p. 4t; 14I. 3§31: "And no person shall throw into the rivers and lagoons, at any time of the year (even if it is outside the said three months of breeding), mockery (1), barbasco (2), cocca (3), lime, or any other material with which to kill the fish. And whoever does so, being a nobleman or squire, or from there upwards, for the first time is degraded one year to Africa, and pays three thousand kings. And for the second time the said penalty of money and banishment shall be doubled: And so for all the times that it is understood, or proven to him. And if he is of lesser quality, he shall be publicly beaten with a barago and nailed, and for any other time that he is caught, or it is proved to him, there shall be the same penalties: and he shall be degraded from the place where he is a resident, and ten leagues around for a period of

legislation, when transported to Brazil, a colony characterized by its abundance of water, was not observed, despite being in force throughout the colonial period[34] . It should also be noted that colonial Brazil was the place where the sentences of banishment would be carried out for some of the environmental offenses, a fact that removed a certain coercive power from this device when practiced in the colony itself.

According to Fabio Feldmann, this lack of interest in the subject did not mean an absence of problems, as chroniclers of the time report problems faced in the city of Rio de Janeiro with human supply, pointing out that major works such as the carioca aqueduct, built in the colonial period, and the reforestation of the Tijuca massif, now the Tijuca National Park, were carried out to bring or guarantee water supply.

At the beginning of the century, public authorities began to worry about formulating a legal framework for managing water resources. The first draft of the Water Code dates back to 1907 and was sent to the National Congress, but the legislative process was not completed. The provisional government of Getulio Vargas in 1930 took up this initiative and on July 10, 1934, Decree 24.643 was promulgated, which had the force of law due to the exceptional situation experienced at the time.

In 1994, Fabio Feldmann considered that:

> The Brazilian Water Code is considered internationally to be one of the most complete water laws ever produced. A number of pioneering principles were introduced and followed in the legislation of various countries. Despite being almost sixty years old, its principles remain valid and are only not applied because several of its provisions have not yet been regulated[35] .

A historical analysis of this document shows a clear liberal inspiration, since it allows

---

one year. This is what we have decided, so as not to kill the fish, nor corrupt the waters of the rivers and lagoons, in which the cattle drink". According to Edis Milare, this provision gave rise to the concept of pollution (Direito do ambiente: doutrina, jurisprudencia, glossario. 3. ed. rev., atual. e ampl., Sao Paulo: Editora Revista dos Tribunais, 2004. p. 115).

[34] FELDMANN, Fabio. Constitutional Review and Water Resources. *In:* MILLAR, Agustin A. (editor). Water resources management and the water market. Brasilia: Secretariat of Irrigation, 1994, p. 12.

[35] FELDMANN, Fabio. Review..., 1994, p. 14.

water resources to be appropriated by private individuals and, contrary to the 1988 Constitution (CF/88), still provides for municipal ownership of some watercourses. This legal institute leaves the idea that water only has an economic value insofar as it is included in private property or can be exploited as hydroelectric potential[36] .

Thus, when it comes to national water resources, the legislation has traditionally treated it as if it were a matter for the electricity sector. In fact, the relative abundance has led to a lack of interest in the subject of water resource management. Fabio Feldmann diagnosed: "Brazilians reflect in their habits a great lack of concern about the possibility of water scarcity, as if they were convinced that it was inexhaustible. This reality is reflected in our legal system and in the administrative practices adopted."[37] .

With the awakening to the importance of water resources, especially in the face of the freshwater crisis, they began to be recognized as limited environmental resources on the brink of an unprecedented crisis. This current phase, aimed at formulating a modern national policy for managing water resources, can be considered to have begun with the creation, in 1978, of the Special Committee for Integrated Studies of Hydrographic Basins (CEEIBH), responsible for integrated studies and monitoring the national use of water resources in the hydrographic basins of federal rivers.

A broader discussion of the issue, with the participation of organized segments of Brazilian society, took shape in the Parliamentary Commission of Inquiry - CPI, of the Chamber of Deputies, which examined the use of water resources in Brazil. This effort continued in 1989 with the Foz do Iguagu Charter, issued by the Brazilian Water Resources Association (ABRH).

Since then, the issue of water resources has been discussed on its own agenda.

---

[36] This is why Maria Luiza Machado Granziera explains the constitutional incoherence (CF 1988) of handing over the ownership of water resources to the federal states and at the same time not allowing these federal entities to legislate on the conservation and preservation of this asset.
[37] FELDMANN, Fabio. op. cit., p. 11.

In Brazil, the journey of recognizing the environmental cause and the need to preserve natural resources was given a voice in the 1988 Constitution, which, in an unprecedented way, inaugurated Chapter VI (art. 225) in the constitutional text, which deals exclusively with the environment. With regard to water resources, the Federal Constitution abolished private ownership of water, handing it over to the Union and the States. It also determined the creation of a national water resources management system.

Law 9.433, of January 8, 1997, inaugurated a new way of thinking about water resources in Brazil, recognizing that it is a limited asset, endowed with economic value, as well as indispensable to life, and must therefore be preserved for present and future generations. It should be noted that the principles enshrined in the Dublin Declaration (listed in the previous chapter) have strong repercussions in national legislation, to the extent that they are, for the most part, reproduced in Article 1 of Law 9.433/97.

The Dublin Declaration states that water resources are finite and essential to human life, development and the environment, while Law 9.433/97 recognizes the limitation of water availability in art. 1, inc. II, and the essentiality of resources for life and various economic activities (art. 1, inc. IV, which prescribes that water must meet multiple uses), even establishing, among the various uses, priority for human consumption and animal watering (art. 1, inc. III).

The Dublin Declaration adopts as the ideal management model one that is integrated and participatory; Law 9.433/97 also chooses this model in art. 1, inc. VI.

The third principle of the Dublin Declaration has not been adopted in Brazilian legislation, because art. 225 of the Federal Constitution establishes the joint responsibility of the government and society in general in preserving environmental resources.

Finally, the recognition in Dublin of the economic value of water is brought into Law 9.433/97, through art. 1, inc. II.

Items from Agenda 21, produced in Rio de Janeiro in 1992, are also present in the legal text in various articles[38] , such as the adoption of the unit for managing water resources, which is now the hydrographic basin, and the national information system on water resources.

Following the effort to implement an efficient water resources policy, Law 9.984 of July 17, 2000 was enacted in Brazil, establishing the National Water Agency - ANA. According to a report by Senator Bernardo Cabral:

> The Executive Branch, in sending PLC No. 3/2000, recognizes that, despite all the efforts made by the brilliant teams that ran the Secretariat of Water Resources, it was unable, for institutional, structural and administrative reasons, to face up to the challenge of implementing the National Water Resources Policy and coordinating the National Water Resources Management System on its own. Legitimate recognition from an administrative, constitutional, legal and responsibility point of view[39] .

This agency would then be in a position to implement a modern system for managing these resources. It should be noted that the ANA came into being during the US-inspired legislative movement based on a neoliberal model of economic policy. Through the latter, the provision of certain public services is handed over to private initiative (privatization of the electricity sector, telecommunications, etc.), under the argument of reducing the state apparatus in order to achieve efficiency in the provision of proper state activities. The policy of state regulation of the economic sector providing public services through regulatory agencies was adopted.

The arguments used as grounds for adopting the agency system are: efficiency, which has been incorporated as a guiding principle for public administration (Constitutional

---

[38] Art. 3 of Law 9.4336/97 corresponds to items A., 18.9 and B, 18.24 of Agenda 21. (A. Development and integrated management of water resources. Objectives. 18.9 Integrated management of water resources, including the integration of aspects related to land and water, should be carried out at catchment or sub-catchment level. B. Assessment of water resources Objectives.18.24. Based on the Mar del Plata Action Plan, this program area was extended into the 1990s and beyond with the general objective of ensuring the assessment and forecasting of the quantity and quality of water resources, in order to estimate the total quantity of these resources and their future supply potential, determine their current quality status, forecast possible supply and demand conflicts and provide a scientific database for the rational use of water resources).

[39] National Water Agency - ANA. Brasilia: Senado Federal, 2001, p. 169-170.

Amendment 19/98); political neutrality, in the sense of greater independence from the executive branch[40] ; technical specialization, so that "the old, lax bureaucratic controls over public services, in which political-partisan arguments always prevailed over technical arguments"[41] gave way to regulatory agencies[42] ; and citizen participation in the management of public affairs, as an expression of political pluralism[43] . Regulatory agencies have been created as special regime autarchies, a form that aims to guarantee them greater independence from state power. They are entities created by law for state intervention in the economic domain, regulating a specific sector, including powers of a regulatory nature and to arbitrate disputes between private individuals and subject to a legal regime that ensures their autonomy from the direct administration[44] .

Regulatory agencies are therefore closely linked to the idea of market regulation. According to the doctrine, regulation can take on three meanings: 1) it refers to all forms of state intervention in the economy, including direct participation in the economy; 2) it relates to intervention in the economy in ways other than direct participation in the exercise of activities of this nature, i.e. conditioning, coordinating and disciplining private economic activity; 3) it means only the normative discipline of the economic sector[45] .

Clarissa Sampaio excludes the first definition, because "for an activity to be characterized as regulation, it is necessary for the state to act as an external agent of the

---

[40] DI PIETRO, Maria Sylvia Zanella. Administrative Law. Sao Paulo: Atlas, 2003, p. 400.
[41] MOREIRA NETO, Diogo de Figueiredo. Course in administrative law: introductory part, general part and special part. Rio de Janeiro: Ed. Forense, 2003, p.437.
[42] "The creation of independent regulatory bodies, as stated above, is linked to the need to guarantee the taking of technical decisions, detached from purely political criteria, so the fact that it is recognized that their field of activity is technical by excellence does not mean that their acts are impermeable in relation to the usual forms of control of the Public Administration, especially the jurisdictional one, notwithstanding the limits and peculiarities that the case raises". (SAMPAIO, Clarissa. Legality and regulation. Belo Horizonte: Forum, 2005, p.20.)
[43] MASTRANGELO, Claudio. Regulatory agencies and popular participation. Porto Alegre: Livraria do Advogado, 2005, p.45.
[44] JUSTEN FILHO, Margal. The law of independent regulatory agencies. São Paulo: Dialdtica, 2002, p. 344.
[45] SAMPAIO, Clarissa. Legality...., p.20.

market"[46] .

The most widely accepted definition of regulation is the second, since the third is too restrictive. The author believes that regulation has broader aims than the prevention of dangers, since it seeks to optimize and balance a given sector, the composition of interests, the defense of a more complex system and not the coercive imposition of the general interest inscribed in a rule. It would therefore be wrong to equate policing with regulation[47] . This does not imply that, in the exercise of regulatory activity, police measures cannot be imposed.

Maria Sylvia Zanella Di Pietro classifies agencies into two types:

> a) those that exercise, on the basis of law, typical police power, with the imposition of administrative limitations, provided for by law, supervision, repression; (...)
> b) those that regulate and control the activities that constitute the object of a concession, permit or authorization for a public service (...) or a concession for the exploitation of a public asset (...)[48] ;

The ANA, in this context, was created as a special regime authority that has the function of a federal entity implementing the National Water Resources Policy, covering the competencies listed in Article 4 of Law 9.984/2000. The authority is run by a Board of Directors, made up of five members, appointed by the President of the Republic. The President of the Republic will choose a CEO from among these members.

The members of the board are not chosen by the Federal Senate, as is the case with the ANP and other agencies, revealing that water is still not considered a strategic asset politically.

The term of office of the board members is four years and they must not coincide. During their term of office, board members are prevented from exercising any professional, trade union or political party leadership activities. These measures are designed to prevent political capture by the government and the private sector, by prioritizing the technical aspect of the decisions taken.

---

[46] Ibid., p.21.
[47] Ibid., p.24.
[48] DI PIETRO, Maria Sylvia Zanella. Law ..., p. 403.

There is no prohibition, after the end of the mandate, on carrying out economic activities in the regulated sector, which would leave privileged information obtained during the mandate open to use by the regulated sector.

Another important fact is that unmotivated dismissals are allowed in the first four months, revealing the fragility of the system at the beginning of the term.

The ANA will be advised by a Public Prosecutor's Office.

The revenues for the administration of the autarchy are those set aside in the Union's budget, donations etc (art. 20 of Law 9.984/2000). At this point, the ANA is particularly important, as it has financial independence from the central political power, to the extent that the funds earned from charging for the use of water resources subject to a grant can be used to manage the National Water Resources Management System (art. 21 of Law 9.984/2000).

The majority of the staff is made up of temporary and commissioned employees (well over 200 commissioned positions - art. 18 and 18-A of Law 9.984/2000). This is detrimental to the ANA's impartiality in the decision-making process, since the technical staff, if not permanent, is easily co-opted by the private sector and the government itself.

The ANA was created to implement the National Water Resources Policy within its sphere of activity. The competencies contained in Article 4 of the aforementioned legal diploma describe deliberative, consultative, normative, supervisory and policing functions.

According to this law, it can be concluded that the ANA's activities are much more focused on preserving water resources. Items I to V, X to XV and XVII of art. 4 deserve to be highlighted, as they are directly and indirectly related to policing and inspection activities, as competencies to implement national policy instruments, the essence of which is conservation. This becomes even more evident when one analyzes the law that created the ANP and the National Oil Policy, whose function is clearly aimed at guaranteeing the market and free competition, so that this agency intervenes in the market to regulate economic dominance along the lines of the second meaning given to the term regulation. It is interesting to note that both the ANP and the ANA have their activities functionalized around a public good, but the economic exploitation of oil has always been in evidence, while it is only today, in the face of threats of water scarcity, that water is recognized as a good of economic value. The normative powers attributed to the ANA show that its function is much more the exercise of police power (like the ANS, ANVISA, etc.) than the regulation of economic activity (like the ANP, ANATEL, etc.).

Chapter 3

Modeling water resource management in foreign law.

3.1 French model. 3.2. German model. 3.3. Spanish model.

Whenever we are faced with a common problem in different legal systems, we are interested in knowing how others have solved it, in order to compare it with our own institutions and learn about the possibilities of foreign experience, in the light of current law or the prospects for change.

When it comes to issues subject to constitutional treatment, however, it is imperative to work with due caution, scrutinizing the entire Constitution, through a careful compatibility test, to find out how far it is possible to transpose doctrinal understandings agreed in the light of foreign legal texts, within the exact limits of the semantic fabric of the Constitution. And this is exactly what is happening in the study of the interaction between tax and environmental competences[49] .

3.1. Frank model.

The French model was created in 1964, through French Law No. 64-1245, of

---

[49] TORRES, Heleno Taveira. The relationship between constitutional tax and environmental competences - the limits of so-called "environmental taxes". In: TORRES, Heleno Taveira (Org.). Direito Tributario Ambiental. Sao Paulo: Malheiros, 2005, p. 96-97.

December 16, 1964, which deals with the regime and distribution of water, as well as combating water pollution. The aim of this law was to restore water quality and adopt a more balanced and sustainable policy.

This legal diploma divided the French territory into six management units (hydrographic basins). Each management unit is made up of a basin committee and a water agency, both of which manage and collect the fees ("redevance") for the services provided.

Most of this law was repealed by *Ordonnance* 2000-914 of September 18, 2000, Law 92-3 of January 3, 1992 and the Environmental Code, but the structure adopted was maintained.

Thus, the main bodies of the French management system are the Basin Committees and the Water Agencies (Environment Code).

The French model is brought into this discussion because it served as an inspiration for the Brazilian model. The Basin Committees, through their manager (mayor), have the task of implementing and coordinating the State's policy on the policing and management of water resources, in order to maintain the unity and coherence of the State's deconcentrated actions (Environment Code). It is known as the water parliament, as it is a body that seeks agreement between those who decide on the water policy to be applied in the corresponding basin. The Basin Committee is made up of members representing the state (20% of its membership) and elected local representatives and water users (80%).

Water agencies are public administrative establishments, endowed with civil personality and financial autonomy. They are responsible for facilitating the various actions of common interest to the basin or basin group, carrying out studies, research and works of common interest to the basins, as well as serving as the administrative body of the water resources system, insofar as they manage the financial resources collected from the "redevance". Each agency is managed by a board of directors made up of representatives from the government, the local population and users.

Participatory management of water resources brings legitimacy to the decisions made within water management bodies. It's a matter of bringing individuals into the public sphere, giving a voice to those directly interested in the functioning of the bodies.

3.2. German model.

The Ministry for the Environment, Nature Conservation and Nuclear Safety is responsible for coordinating matters relating to water resources; the Ministry for Economic Affairs, for its part, is responsible for controlling water supply and the water industry, while the Federal Office for the Environment is responsible for protecting water resources as an environmental asset[50] .

There is a cohesive approach to the economic and environmental management of water resources, with a view to avoiding a watertight and separate treatment of the issue by various public bodies, a situation that is very similar to the institutionalization of the Water System. National Water Resources in Brazil, as will be detailed below.

In Germany, there are no federal government bodies to enforce legislation, and the states are responsible for executing federal laws as their own affairs. However, the Federal Government is responsible for controlling the legality of the acts of state bodies, but the "exercise of police power with regard to inspection and the granting of licenses is the responsibility of the states, including in the area of water management and protection"[51] .

Andreas Krell explains that, due to the large number of small municipalities (around

---

[50] KRELL, Andreas J. Basic Instruments for the Management and Protection of Water Resources in Germany. In: Revista Brasileira de Direito Ambiental, ano 2, v. 5, Sao Paulo: Fiuza, jan./mar., 2006, p. 46.
[51] KRELL, Andreas J. Instrumentos ..., p. 46.

13,500), it was not possible to maintain a vast number of bodies and offices to deal with the many competencies, and so the creation of inter-municipal and inter-governmental cooperation bodies, called Kreis (made up of an average of 20 to 30 municipalities), evolved. The Kreis is both a unit of the state administration and an association of municipalities.

The powers of the Kreis are based on the principle of subsidiarity, according to which higher authorities can only take on tasks and services that smaller authorities are unable to perform[52] . Andreas Krell explains, with regard to the management of water resources:

> A wide range of tasks related to the management and protection of water resources fall to the Kreis as a unit of action of the state administration, such as inspection, granting of water concessions and the execution of water plans. In addition, some states have their own specialized technical departments, which are not part of the Kreis structure, but report directly to the State Secretariat for the Environment. Kreis also acts as an inter-municipal association for the construction and maintenance of wastewater treatment plants[53] .

For a long time, Germany did not have specific water legislation, although water law was one of the oldest branches of German environmental law, which was initially based on customary law, then on private law and finally on public law. Subsequently, several states issued regulations on the use of surface water, irrigation and flood protection. In 1957, the Federal Water Management Act *(Wasserhaushaltsgesetz* - WHG) regulated "almost all circumstances that could lead to a reduction in the quantity or degradation of existing water. The WHG has been amended several times and was enacted again in 2002."[54] . This law regulates surface, coastal and subterranean waters and implements many principles of environmental law:

> the principle of prevention through the explicit attempt to avoid certain burdens and damage to water resources from the outset. The principle of cooperation is the ideological basis for allowing water associations administrative autonomy and for creating the figure of the 'company officer' *(Betriesbeauftragter) for* water protection (arts. 21-21g WHG), obliging larger companies to hire a specialist to monitor internal

---

[52] Ibid., p. 46.
[53] Ibid., p. 49.
[54] KRELL, Andreas J. Instrumentos ..., p. 50.

compliance with environmental legislation and to advocate integrating the goal of environmental protection into company policy by promoting research and the development of innovative processes and products. The principle of responsibility ('polluter pays'), in turn, is contemplated by the requirement to use the 'best available technique' in the treatment of effluents, which leads to higher operating costs for the respective issuer. The principle of 'integral water management' also prevails, recognizing that problems in this area cannot be solved solely through the use of traditional administrative sanction instruments[55] .

In 1976, the WHG underwent changes, introducing into the legal system a standardization of the criteria for issuing water grants and water quality targets. It also introduced various planning instruments, such as sewage disposal plans, regional water plans and water source protection plans[56] . An effluent tax was also introduced as a strategy to reduce river pollution caused by wastewater.

According to Thomas Zumbroich, this regulation, based on the Water Reserves Act, obliges each member state of the Federal Republic of Germany to collect a tax on the direct emission of water containing polluting substances. [57]

In a nutshell, here's the formula: the higher the load of toxic substances, the higher the amount to be paid by industries and municipalities for the emission of wastewater into rivers and streams. The money raised is invested mainly in improving wastewater treatment facilities and in sewage and sanitation services. Today, the success of this model can be seen in the effective improvement of water quality in almost all rivers in Germany[58] .

3.3. Spanish model

Spain's Water Law (Law 29 of August 2, 1985) recognizes water as a scarce resource,

---

[55] Ibid., p. 50-51.
[56] Ibid., p. 51.

indispensable for life and for the exercise of most economic activities, irreplaceable, vulnerable and susceptible to multiple uses. Law 29/85 also recognizes that water resources must be treated as a unit, and that the management of surface water cannot be distinguished from that of groundwater.

This law breaks new ground in the Spanish legal system by abolishing the possibility of private individuals appropriating underground water resources, in accordance with the repealed water legislation (Law of June 13, 1879). The preamble to this law is emphatic:

> On the other hand, the current Water Law of June 13, 1879, a model in its kind and in its time, cannot respond to the requirements raised by the
>
> [57]   ZUMBROICH, Thomas. The Guideline..., p. 25.
> [58]   Ibid, p. 26.
>
> new territorial organization of the State, born of the 1978 Constitution, the profound transformations experienced by society, technological advances, the pressure of demand and the growing awareness of ecology and improving the quality of life. Good proof of this is the legislative frontier that has been enacted to date, with varying levels of regulation, in its attempt, sometimes unsuccessful, to accommodate changing socio-economic, cultural, political, geographical and even survival circumstances, as in some cases of overexploitation or serious contamination of aquifers.
>
> A new legislation on the subject is therefore essential, one that takes full advantage of the undoubted successes of previous legislation and includes traditional institutions for regulating the rights of irrigators, an example of which is the Valencian Water Court, but which takes into account the changes that have taken place and, in particular, the new autonomous configuration of the State, so that the exercise of the competences of the different Administrations takes place within the obligatory framework of collaboration, in order to achieve a rational use and adequate protection of the resource[57] .

The Spanish management system is governed by the principle of unity of management, respecting the hydrographic unit, recognizing the economic value of water and the participation of users in the management system. Management will also be deconcentrated, decentralized, coordinated and effective (art. 13).

This law provides for the following management instruments: licensing, plans and "canones de vertidos". The structure of the Spanish system includes the National Water

---

[57] SPAIN. Water Law. Madrid: Ministry of Public Works and Urban Planning, 1990, p. 70.

Council, an advisory body made up of representatives of the State, the Autonomous Communities and professional and economic organizations related to the different uses of water (art. 17). There is also a provision for user communities (art. 73), which makes it possible for users to participate in the Spanish state's water policy.

In the Spanish model, water taxation is subject to what legislation and doctrine refer to as canons ("canon por ocupacion del dominio publico", "canon de vertido", "canon de regulation"). Tulio Rosembuj explains:

> The very name 'canon' induces a notable ambiguity. The canon is a non-existent tax figure... The canon is the price for the creation of specific and appropriate powers for the private or communal use of a natural resource, in this case water. La Administration obtiene una compensation porque, ejercando las potestades que le confiere el derecho, faculta al particular para el disfrute o aprovechamiento[58] .

Herrera Molina and Carbajo Vasco recognize, however, that canons or charges have a tax nature. In their words: "La utilization del dominio publico ambiental constituye un campo idoneo para el estabelecimiento de tasas (a nuestro juicio esta es la naturaleza del nuevo canon de control de vertidos previsto en la Ley de Aguas"[59] .

---

[58] TORRES, Ricardo Lobo. The taxation of public services in the state of the risk society. *In:* TORRES, Ricardo Lobo (Coord.) Servicos Publicos e Direito Tributario. Sao Paulo: Quartier Latin, 2005, p. 139.
[59] MOLINA, Pedro Manuel Herrera and VASCO, Domingo Carbajo. Conceptual, Constitutional and Community Framework for Ecological Taxation. In: TORRES, Heleno Taveira (Org.). Direito Tributario Ambiental. Sao Paulo: Malheiros, 2005, p. 190.

Chapter 4

Constitutional water regime.

4.1 Legislative competence. 4.2. Material competence. 4.3.
Ownership of water resources

4.1. Legislative competence.

Water resources gained a new constitutional approach with the Federal Constitution of
198 8[60] , since the constituent legislator not only recognized them as a strategic environmental
resource for the energy sector[61] , giving them economic treatment, but also moved away from a
classic patrimonialist optic and began to conceive of them as a diffuse good, establishing a
shared socio-environmental responsibility between society and the state.

The constituent legislator maintained the tradition started by the 1934 Constitution, in
the sense that legislation on water was left privately to the Union (art. 22, inc. IV). This
maintains the criticized fragmentation of the environment, which allows the patrimonialization
of environmental goods and their appropriation by the state, disregarding the fact that
environmental goods are part of the diffuse heritage of society[62] . On the other hand, this

---

[60] "Environmentalism has become a topic of great importance in the most recent Constitutions. It deliberately
enters them as a fundamental right of the human person, not as a simple aspect of the attribution of organs or
public entities as occurred in older Constitutions". (SILVA, Jose Afonso da. Constitutional Environmental Law.
Sao Paulo: Malheiros Editores, 2002, p. 43)

[61] Since the 1934 Constitution, the Brazilian state has adopted the technique of privately assigning the power to
legislate on water resources to the Union.

[62] Beyond the classic distinction between public and private property, the concept of diffuse property stands out.
For a given analysis, this heritage is made up of assets that belong neither to private individuals nor to the state,
although there is a tendency to publicize the ownership of some diffuse assets. Diffuse heritage is not demarcated
by the sense of ownership, but by the degree of importance for the survival of this and future generations, and
encompasses a significant number of assets. The ownership that materializes in the notarial system is not central
to the reading of this type of property. Diffuse assets are not demarcated by the sense of exclusive ownership;
their logic is different. The fundamental notes are inclusion and sharing.

35

provision has the salutary effect of, at least in the case of water, working with the geographical unit of the asset (hydrographic basin) and considering the sharing of hydro-environmental impacts in the hydrographic basins, disseminating a uniform treatment of the issue throughout the Brazilian state.

What the law aims to protect is the quality of the environment as a function of the quality of life. It can be said that there are two objects of protection in this case: an immediate one, which is the quality of the environment; and an intermediate one, which is the health, well-being and safety of the population, which has been summarized in the expression "quality of life". The quality of the environment thus becomes a good that the law recognizes and protects as environmental heritage[63] .

The fragmentation of the environment is a step towards the patrimonialization of environmental goods, as Jose Robson da Silva argues:

> Unavailable rights are integrated into the market through different stratagems, moral heritage is valued in pecuniary terms, the products of donated blood are marketed, eyes go to a bank and those who can afford them skip the queue for organ transplants - the market imposes itself on people and the environment. Nature is divided, fragmented and patrimonialized. In this context, a tough clash is taking place between the critical doctrine, which is oriented towards the repersonalization of the law and going beyond the anthropocentric, and the liberal doctrine, which advocates the complete patrimonialization of nature.
>
> The paradox of this process of patrimonialization is that the law enshrined in the Brazilian Constitution of 1988 is refractory to it. In the Constitution, the exact opposite is the case, since the deprivatization, protection of human dignity and environmental balance are the hallmarks[64] .

It should be emphasized that considerable doctrine[65] points out that the legislator's

---

[63] SILVA, Josě Afonso da. Environmental Law..., p. 81-82.
[64] SILVA, Josě Robson da. Paradigma Biocentrico: do patrimonio privado ao patrimonio ambiental. Rio de Janeiro: Renovar, 2002, p. 279.
[65] GERALDES, Andre Gustavo de Almeida. Legal protection of water sources. Sao Paulo: Editora Juarez de Oliveira, 2004, p. 87-88. GRAFF, Ana Claudia Bento. State protection of water. In: Waters - legal and environmental aspects. Vladimir Passos de Freitas (Org.), Curitiba: Jurua, 2001, p. 56-61. POMPEU, Cid Tomanik. Recursos hidricos na Constituigao de 1988, Revista de Direito Administrativo, n.186, Rio de Janeiro: Renovar, Oct/Dec/1991, p. 22.

choice stems from the need to control hydroenergetic potential[66] and that, in doing so, he has created a paradox: the Union's exclusive competence to legislate on water and the competence of each federal entity to legislate on public property in its domain, with Granziera understanding that

> If states were forbidden the power to lay down rules on property under their control, there would be a gap in the law, since the Union would not be able to legislate in administrative matters on property that does not belong to it.
>
> The way to resolve the impasse was to understand that the competence to legislate on water, in a general sense and which belongs to the Union, should not be confused with the ability of each Brazilian political entity - the Union, States, Federal District and Municipalities - to establish administrative rules on the assets that are under their respective dominion, this term being understood as custody and administration[67].

Although we recognize that an analysis of these rules of jurisdiction, as proposed, may suggest an apparent antinomy, we do not see how this conflict can be resolved by imposing rules similar to the technique applied to matters subject to concurrent legislation (general legislation falling within the competence of the Union and specific legislation falling within the competence of the states). Indeed, if the constituent legislator had wanted to establish concurrent legislation on water, he would not have included it in the list in art. 22, but in the list in art. 24.

Therefore, the forgone conclusion is that the Union is not solely responsible for legislating on general rules, as proposed by the author; on the contrary, it can legislate exhaustively on the matter, if it sees fit and convenient. However, it is allowed for the Union, through a complementary law, to authorize the states to legislate on specific issues (sole paragraph of art. 22)[68]. However, this legislative delegation has not been drawn up to date.

---

[66] "This rule, which was extremely centralizing, was suitable for the control of hydroelectric potential, which is granted by the Union, which is also competent to legislate privately on energy." (GRANZIERA, Maria Luiza Machado. Direito de aguas: disciplina juridica das aguas doces. Sao Paulo: Atlas, 2001, p. 67).

[67] Ibid., p. 67.

[68] In the opposite direction, it is understood that the exclusive competence to legislate on water, attributed to the Union, refers only to the creation of the national system of water resources and the definition of granting criteria

It should be noted that, for legislative delegation, the formal (complementary law), material (the generality of the matter cannot be delegated, but only a specific point of the matter) and implicit (in the sense that the delegation cannot establish preference between the federated entities) requirements must be met.

In fact, we don't see any inconsistency or paradox, because there is no incompatibility in maintaining legislation on the Union's exclusive competence, which allows for unified treatment of the matter[69] , and at the same time handing over the management of the asset to more than one federal entity, a fact that allows for decentralization. By way of illustration, it should be remembered that procedural legislation is the exclusive preserve of the Union and the management of justice is entrusted to the judicial powers of each state and federal government.

It should be borne in mind that the Federal Constitution, when it inaugurated the Brazilian legal order in 1988, established that the management of water resources would be decentralized and handed over to the states and the Union, but the legal regime of this environmental asset, as an instrument of environmental policy, would be established by national legislation drawn up by the Union.

It is true that there are no concurrent legislative competences in the area of water, but there are certain matters attributed to concurrent competence which, when dealt with in a specific normative instrument, can touch on the subject, such as the competence to legislate on nature conservation, the defense of the soil and natural resources, the protection of the environment, the control of pollution (art. 24, inc. VI), liability for environmental damage (art.

---

for federal waters. "The reference there is to the management of water resources, the ownership of which belongs to the Union, since it would be unconstitutional to interpret the term 'water resources' to include those belonging to the federal states, which are the *dominus;* consequently, the definition of the 'criteria for granting their use', referred to in the constitutional text mentioned, concerns only federal waters." (MUKAI, Toshio. Direito Ambiental..., p. 53).

[69] "There is a broad scope of the Union's normative power, which must be used so that state legislations do not create discriminatory rules or stimulate different and even antagonistic policies on the use of water" (MACHADO, Paulo Affonso Leme. Water Resources - Brazilian and International Law. Sao Paulo: Malheiros Ediotres, 2002, p. 19).

24, inc. XII) and the protection and defense of health (art. 24, inc. XII). 24, inc. VI), liability

for environmental damage (art. 24, inc. VIII) and the protection and defense of health[70] (art.

24, inc. XII). In fact, as it is an environmental asset, water ends up being affected by

legislation protecting natural resources. Despite this interconnection of themes, the Federal

Supreme Court tends to recognize that private competences override concurrent competences,

which implies that the matter dealt with by the Union will take precedence over that dealt with

by the other federal entities[71] . Paulo de Bessa Antunes gives an example:

> When legislating on mines, for example, the Union is exercising all of its competence
> over the matter, including environmental competence, adopting the criterion that the
> accessory follows the principal, i.e. concurrent competence will only be exercised to
> the extent that it conforms to the federal standard defined in the exclusive
> competence area. No state or municipal rule can, by way of environmental protection,
> go so far as to make it impossible to carry out an activity as defined by the Union in
> the exclusive use of its powers. This is a parameter that must be followed in any and
> all matters that, when dealt with within the Union's exclusive jurisdiction, have

---

[70] Health has an immediate correlation with the quality of water resources, as numerous diseases can be caused or spread through water.

[71] In her opinion in Adi 2396- MC, Justice Ellen Gracie clarifies that "In the CF/88 system, as in the previous ones, the general legislative competence belongs to the Federal Union. The residual or implicit competence belongs to the States, which 'can legislate on matters that are not reserved to the Union and that do not concern the proper administration of the Municipalities, as far as their peculiar interests are concerned' (Representation No. 1.153-4/RS, vote of Mim. Moreira Alves)". Thus, with due regard for the differences highlighted by the Minister in terms of the content of the wording between the 1967 and 1988 Constitutions, it is worth collating an excerpt from the vote delivered by the Minister in Representation 1.153-4 - RS, which demonstrates the prevalence of federal legislation over state legislation and the criteria established for making such an assessment, which, in the field of water resources, are fully applicable to this day: "Finally, attention should be drawn to the circumstance that, when a given matter is complex, in the sense that it involves aspects of which one falls within the exclusive competence of the Federal Union and the other within the supplementary competence of the Member States, the discipline of this complex matter falls exclusively within the exclusive competence of the Union, since exclusive competence is absolute, and therefore cannot be directly or indirectly removed, as would occur if, in the complex matter to be legislated, the value of the aspects at stake were examined, in order to make one of them prevail, and consequently make this matter fall within the exclusive competence of the union or the non-cumulative concurrent competence between it and the member states. This is why, when it comes to the production, marketing and consumption of medicines - a complex matter, since it involves international trade and interstate trade, as well as public health - it is exclusively up to the union to impose restrictions on their production, marketing and consumption throughout the national territory, on the grounds that they are harmful to health. The Union would not have this power - which it has never been denied - if, between the exclusive competence to legislate on foreign and interstate trade and the concurrent competence to legislate on general rules for the defense and protection of health, preference could be given to the latter in order to place this matter in the field of this current competence of general principles, which would prevent the Union from not only having exclusive power to judge what was harmful to health, but also from being able to say specifically whether or not this or that medicine was harmful to health, and therefore prohibited from being produced, marketed and consumed. The distinction between exclusive competence and concurrent competence was not made in view of the intrinsic value of the materials that constitute the object of one or the other (health represents a higher value than foreign and interstate trade), but rather in view of the interest of the federation, which requires that certain materials, whatever aspects they may have (such as foreign or interstate trade in goods that may harm health), have the same discipline throughout the national territory, which is only possible through the attribution of exclusive competence to the Union to legislate on them".

environmental repercussions (concurrent jurisdiction). It is possible to say that exclusive jurisdiction exercises a right of pre-emption over concurrent and even common jurisdiction, whenever a point of contact is identified between them. What is made explicit here, of course, is not the author's personal desire, but the way in which judicial and administrative practice has resolved the issues: with greater centralization[72] .

The Federal Supreme Court has also established that states cannot legislate until the complementary law referred to in the sole paragraph of art. 22 of the Charter of the Republic has been enacted[73] .

Thus, although there is an apparent antinomy in this field, the conflict will be resolved in the specific case by applying the criteria of specialty[74] and hierarchy. Indeed, when national environmental legislation and national water legislation conflict, the latter should prevail, even if it predates the former. When state legislation on the environment, which incidentally deals with water, and national water legislation conflict, the rule produced by the Union should always prevail.

It should be pointed out that, in matters of concurrent jurisdiction, the Federal Supreme Court also recognizes a certain overlap between the legislation drawn up by the Union and that of the other federal entities. Practice shows that legislation, which should be general, often goes into such detail that, even though the states draw up specific legislation, they end up clashing with legislation drawn up as a general rule. According to Paulo de Bessa Antunes, this is due to the lack of a federal law on general rules (art. 24, §3, of the Federal Constitution), a fact that prevents the Supreme Court from adopting reliable parameters to indicate, in specific

---

[72] ANTUNES, Paulo de Bessa. Environmental Law. Editora Lumen Juris: Rio de Janeiro, 2006, p. 75

[73] EMENTA: DIRECT ACTION FOR UNCONSTITUTIONALITY. LAW NO. 7.723/99 OF THE STATE OF RIO GRANDE DO NORTE. INSTALLMENT PAYMENT OF TRAFFIC FINES. FORMAL UNCONSTITUTIONALITY. (1) This Court, in repeated pronouncements, has held that the Constitution of Brazil has conferred exclusively on the Union the power to legislate on traffic, and it is certain that the Member States cannot, until the advent of the complementary law provided for in the sole paragraph of article 22 of the CB/88, legislate on the matters listed in the precept. (ADI 2432-RN, Rel. Min. Eros Grau, DJU 26/8/2005, p. 5, republished DJU 23/9/2005, p. 7). Precedents: ADI/MC n. 2328, Reporting Justice Mauricio Correa, DJ of 15.12.2000; ADI n. 2101, Reporting Justice Mauricio Correa, DJ of 05.10.2001; ADI 1704, Reporting Justice Carlos Velloso, DJ of 20.09.2000; ADI 2101, Reporting Justice Mauricio Correa, DJ of 25.10.2001; ADI 1592, Reporting Justice Moreira Alves, DJ of 09.05.2003).

[74] The criterion of specialty applies insofar as we understand that the fragmentation of the environmental good requires specific treatment of water resources.

cases, which state legislations are in violation of the general law. According to the aforementioned author, there is a tendency for the Supreme Court to identify federal legislation, in its entirety, with a general rule[75] . For this reason, it is not uncommon for state legislation, produced on the basis of concurrent competence, to be declared unconstitutional because it violates federal law.

These statements are illustrated by the fact that the Federal Supreme Court believes that supplementary legislation is responsible for filling in the gaps left by federal legislation, without diametrically opposing it[76] , in a way that ends up showing an overestimation of the scope and breadth that federal legislation can reach.

Therefore, the thematic interconnection between water and the environment, which

---

[75] ANTUNES, Paulo de Bessa. Law ..., p. 81.

[76] DIRECT ACTION FOR UNCONSTITUTIONALITY. LAW NO. 2.210/01, OF THE STATE OF MATO GROSSO DO SUL. INFRINGEMENT OF ARTICLES 22, IE XII; 25, § 1; 170, CAPUT, II AND IV; 1; 18 AND 5 *CAPUT,* II AND LIV. INEXISTENCE. INFRINGEMENT OF THE UNION'S CONCURRENT LEGISLATIVE COMPETENCE TO ISSUE GENERAL RULES ON PRODUCTION AND CONSUMPTION, ENVIRONMENTAL PROTECTION AND POLLUTION CONTROL AND HEALTH PROTECTION AND DEFENSE. ARTICLE 24, V, VIE XII AND §§ 1 AND 2 OF THE FEDERAL CONSTITUTION. It is not up to this Court to give the final word on the technical-scientific properties of the element in question and the risks of its use for the health of the population. Studies in this area are continuing and their conclusions should guide the actions of the health authorities. The Supreme Court's jurisdiction is limited to verifying whether there is an inadmissible contrast between the law under examination and the constitutional parameter. Since it is possible for this Supreme Court, based on the facts narrated in the initial decision, to verify the occurrence of an attack on constitutional provisions other than those indicated in the initial decision, it can be seen that in determining a ban on the manufacture, entry, sale and storage of asbestos or asbestos-based products intended for civil construction, the State of Mato Grosso do Sul has exceeded the scope of its concurrent competence to legislate on production and consumption (art. 24, V). 24, V); environmental protection and pollution control (art. 24, VI); and health protection (art. 24, XII). Law No. 9.055/95 makes extensive provisions on all aspects concerning the production and industrial use, transportation and marketing of chrysotile asbestos. The contested legislation falls far outside the scope of supplementary legislation, which is expected to fill gaps or loopholes left by federal legislation, not to make provisions in diametric opposition to it. This is the understanding that the Supreme Court has expressed when faced with cases of concurrent legislative competence. Precedents: ADI 903/MG-MC and ADI 1.980/PR-MC, both written by the eminent Minister Celso de Mello. Direct action of unconstitutionality whose request is partially granted to declare the unconstitutionality of article 1 and its §§ 1, 2 and 3, of article 2, of article 3 and §§ 1 and 2 and of the sole paragraph of article 5, all of Law No. 2.210/01, of the State of Mato Grosso do Sul. (ADI 2396).
EMENTA: CONSTITUTIONAL. DIRECT ACTION. INJUNCTION. WORK OR ACTIVITY POTENTIALLY HARMFUL TO THE ENVIRONMENT. PRIOR ENVIRONMENTAL IMPACT STUDY. In view of the broad terms of item IV of paragraph 1 of art. 225 of the Federal Charter, the argument that the state rule which exempts prior environmental impact studies in the case of afforestation or reforestation areas for business purposes is unconstitutional is legally relevant. Even if we were to admit the possibility of such a restriction, the law that could make it possible would fall within the competence of the federal legislature, since it is up to the federal legislature to regulate, through general rules, the conservation of nature and the protection of the environment (art. 24, inc. VI, of the FC), and it is also not possible to consider the legislative competence referred to in par. 3. of art. 24 of the Federal Charter, since the latter seeks to fill regulatory gaps to meet local peculiarities, which are absent in this case. Preliminary injunction granted (ADI 1086 MC/SC).

would apparently justify the exercise of supplementary legislative powers by the states and the Federal District - with regard to protecting water, combating pollution of this asset, liability for damage to water resources and the defense and protection of health caused by water - would be restricted to filling in gaps or loopholes left by federal legislation and provided that it did not contradict it. In practice, federal legislation on water would override any state or district legislation, even if it was drawn up within the scope of concurrent competence, because the constitutional interpretation made by the Federal Supreme Court prevents the state, using its supplementary competence, from formulating a discipline that ends up ruling out the application of federal rules of a general nature. This ends up confirming, even if any polemic could be raised with regard to concurrent competences, that, in water matters, the Union's legislation has an almost dictatorial character[77] .

It is forgivable to conclude that, in water matters, the states, the Federal District and the municipalities must faithfully comply with the water legislation, because there is no complementary law authorizing the states to legislate on specific points of the matter, a fact that prevents these entities from exercising their legislative competence, and because, in practice, even when the issue touches on matters delegated to concurrent competence, the general law takes real precedence over any local legislation.

Given this constitutional framework, one has to wonder about the constitutionality of the water laws drawn up by the states which, at first glance, in view of this constitutional dynamic, could be considered unconstitutional because they would violate the Union's exclusive competence to legislate on the matter.

---

[77] A similar conclusion is reached to the stance adopted by the Federal Supreme Court in ADI 3035 with regard to genetically modifiable organisms: EMENTA: Direct action of unconstitutionality filed against Paraná state law no. 14.162, of October 27, 2003, which establishes a ban on the cultivation, manipulation, importation, industrialization and commercialization of genetically modified organisms. 2) Alleged violation of the following constitutional provisions: art. 1; art. 22, items I, VII, VI; art. 24, I and VI; art. 25 and art. 170 cap. (2) Alleged violation of the following constitutional provisions: art. 1; art. 22, items I, VII, X and XI; art. 24, I and VI; art. 25 and art. 170, *caput,* item IV and sole paragraph. (3) Offense against the exclusive competence of the Union and the constitutional rules relating to matters of concurrent legislative competence. 4. action upheld.

In fact, in the current regulatory framework, the states and the Federal District cannot legislate on water and, when there is an interconnection with the matters listed in art. 24, state legislation must respect the precedence of federal legislation. In short, the states and the Federal District must currently faithfully observe the Water Law (Law 9.433/97) and the Water Code (insofar as it is still in force). Moreira Alves' link cannot be repeated enough:

> The distinction between exclusive competence and concurrent competence was not made with regard to the intrinsic value of the matters that constitute the object of one or the other (...), but rather in view of the interest of the federation, which requires that certain matters, whatever their aspects (...), have the same discipline throughout the national territory, which is only possible through the attribution of exclusive competence to the Union to legislate on them[78] .

In fact, water needs to be dealt with on the basis of centralized legislation, because only in this way is it possible to respect the geographical unity that imposes the sharing of hydro-environmental impacts in hydrographic basins, i.e. any alteration at one point in the basin could fatally affect another, even if it is far away. It is not uncommon, for example, for the lack of sanitation programs in one municipality to affect another more drastically, insofar as it ends up polluting its groundwater. Therefore, the Union can, if it wishes, subject "all waters to strict public control, especially with a view to their preservation and legal protection against all forms of degradation"[79] .

However, the Union has chosen to draw up legislation that makes it possible for federated entities to cooperate in conserving and preserving water resources. Law 9.433/97 allows for decentralized and participatory management and expressly coordinates the action of the state and federal public authorities (articles 29 and 30), but this does not mean that the Union has handed over the legislative function to the state to carry out fully or partially; on the contrary, what this legal diploma has done is establish a form of federated cooperation for the

---

[78] STF: Representation 1.513-RS.
[79] SILVA, ■ГсБё Afonso da. Environmental Law..., p. 126.

respective entities to exercise the power to police water.

In short, state regulations on water are subordinated exclusively to the discipline proposed by the Union. In fact, not even the discipline of land use by state law to protect water sources in metropolitan regions is admissible, contrary to what Tc3ë Afonso da Silva[80][81] states, citing, as a reference, the decision handed down in Representation 1.007[83,] pointed out in Paulo Afonso Leme's work[82] . From a careful reading of this Representation, the Federal Supreme Court unanimously - still under the 1967 Constitution, which kept water legislation under the exclusive competence of the Union[83] - declared the unconstitutionality of the São Paulo laws that dealt with water.

The following are excerpts from the winning vote of Justice Cordeiro Guerra:

> Therefore, it must be admitted that the rules of São Paulo's legislation, which are the subject of this representation, by regulating the use of springs, streams, reservoirs and other water resources in the state, have invaded the Union's field of legislative competence, consequently violating the Constitution, as well as establishing priorities other than the purposes recognized by the Federal Constitution, conflict with it, and cannot stand.
>
> (..)
>
> In so deciding, I do not deny, in theory, the administrative police power of all state entities in the preservation of the environment, but I condition it to the limits of their territory and the constitutionally established legislative competence[84] .

Finally, it is important to address the competence to regulate the exercise of water policing powers.

It is interesting to note that, already under the previous Constitution, legislative

---

[80] Ibid., p. 123.

[81] EMENTA: Laws n. 898, of December 18, 1975 and n. 1.172, of November 17, 1976, which, respectively, regulate the use of land for the protection of water sources, water courses and reservoirs and other water resources of interest to the metropolitan region of Greater Sao Paulo and delimit the areas of protection to water sources, water courses and reservoirs, and make other provisions. Unconstitutionality of the sole paragraph of Article 5 and item IV of Article 11 of Law 898, and of item I of Article 2, Article 8 and its paragraphs and items I, III and IV of Article 9 of Law 172. The defense of the environment must be exercised with respect for the legislative competence of the Federal Union. Representation upheld.

[82] MACHADO, Paulo Affonso Leme. Resources ..., p. 120.

[83] 1967 Constitution: Article 8 - The Union is responsible for: XVII - legislating on: i) water, electricity and telecommunications.

[84] STF: Representation 1.007.

competence in water matters and competence to regulate police power clashed. In

Representation 1.007, the State of Sao Paulo's motivation clearly demonstrates the

controversy, when the then Governor of the State of Sao Paulo, Egydio Martins, states that the

contested laws were inspired by

> in the overriding public interest of arming the State Administration with the instruments necessary for the effective exercise of police power, with regard to the pollution of water resources in the Metropolitan Region of Greater Sao Paulo (...) the legislation is clearly administrative in nature, with regard to the classification of inland waters[85] .

In its opinion, the Public Prosecutor's Office, in the aforementioned representation, states the following and the

Rapporteur Minister Cordeiro Guerra, on page 28 of his vote, adopts the following as a basis:

> In fact, although we recognize the high aims contained in the São Paulo laws in question regarding the fight against pollution and the better use of watercourses for the purposes of the human environment, we must verify, however, in view of the constitutional provisions, that they have entered into a specific field of another sphere of competence or, at the very least, have clashed with the federal competence for the exploitation of electric energy services and for legislation on water and energy in general, provided for in art. 8, XV, letter 'b' and XVII, letter 'i'[86] .

On these grounds, Justice Cordeiro Guerra admits the exercise of police power by all

state entities with regard to the preservation of the environment, but restricts it to the limits of

the territory and constitutional competence.

This historical record demonstrates that, even under the 1967 Constitution, the

boundaries separating regulatory legislation for the exercise of police powers to combat

pollution and water legislation were already very tenuous. At the time, the Federal Supreme

Court recognized that water legislation took precedence over the competence to regulate police

powers.

---

[85] STF: Representation 1.007.
[86] 1967 Constitution: Article 8 - The Union is responsible for: XV - exploring, directly or through authorization or concession: b) electric energy services and installations of any origin or nature; XVII - legislating on: i) water, electric energy and telecommunications.

Despite the fact that the constitutional competences in the field of water have not changed, following the global trend of concern for the environment - in order to reconcile economic development with the preservation of the environment, today reflected in the right to sustainable development - the Federal Constitution introduced a new parameter into the national legal system, namely that of co-responsibility (society and public authorities) for the environmental good, so that everyone must seek its preservation and conservation for present and future generations.

On the other hand, it must be recognized that, in terms of private legislation, the Union enjoys real precedence. With regard to water - where the geographical unity of water resources, which imposes the sharing of hydro-environmental impacts, cannot be ignored - it is essential to make a conciliatory reading of the provisions that determine the powers to legislate on water and to regulate police power.

Even because, as Andreas Krell states:

> (...) in practice, the principle that each sphere of government could only apply its own rules was never strictly obeyed. It can be seen that the application of higher legislation has long since become a reality in the administrative procedures of many Brazilian municipalities.[87]

From a traditional point of view, the power to police a given activity is part of the powers of the internal public law body with legislative competence over the subject, since the power to police is a consequence of the competence. Thus, by dividing up the material competences between each federal entity, the Constitution gives them the power to legislate and the power to supervise, respectively[88] . Thus, when the Constitution assigns to the Union the exploration of nuclear services and activities, under the terms of art. 21, inc. XXIII, it also

---

[87] KRELL, Andreas J.. Administrative discretion and environmental protection: the control of undetermined legal concepts and the competence of environmental bodies: a comparative study. Porto Alegre: Livraria do Advogado, 2004, p. 98.

[88] FREITAS, Vladimir Passos de. Administrative law and the environment. 3. ed., 2. tir., Curitiba: Jurua, 2002, p. 88.

assigns respectively the competence to legislate and to supervise .[89]

However, this solution does not resolve the apparent conflict in water matters. In fact, based on the example above, it is easy to see that the development of nuclear activity is not part of environmental heritage, although it can certainly cause irreversible and irreparable damage. Water, on the other hand, is part of the environmental heritage, which is why, under Article 225 of the Federal Constitution, it is affected by the supervisory powers of other federal entities. In this case, is there a split in the sense that, in order to inspect, it is not necessary to legislate on the matter? It seems that case law is moving in this direction.

There seems to be no constitutional impediment to the Union legislating and the other entities applying their legislation to protect the environment and combat pollution. This is Andreas Krell's view:

> The express distinction between legislative powers on the one hand and administrative powers on the other would also make no sense if each political sphere continued to be able to enforce its own rules. The twelve clauses of Article 23 of the Constitution would simply be superfluous if this administrative competence existed only in connection with the respective powers to legislate, as was the case under previous Brazilian constitutions.(...)
> We therefore believe that in Brazil the traditional system of administrative separation has been partially revised by the new Federal Constitution. In the areas listed in art. 23, it is now possible for municipalities to also enforce federal or state regulations when they deem it necessary[90] .

Incidentally, a similar case is being discussed by the Supreme Court in RE 194.704-MG, and this is the direction in which the Court's final decision is heading. In this case, the competence to legislate on traffic and the competence to protect the environment and combat pollution clashed, with Justice Cezar Peluso concluding that "the protection of the environment and the fight against pollution by the municipality could only take place through the application of federal legislation on the matter, notably the National Traffic Code - CNT (...)"[91]

---

[89] Ibid., p. 88.
[90] KRELL, Andreas J.. Discretion..., p. 99.
[91] STF: RE 194.704-MG.

The power to legislate on water would override the power to legislate on environmental protection and pollution. What the other federal entities are allowed to do is, through legislation, organize the public services that make it possible to apply the national protective legislation, in other words, the states can legislate on the organization of the water inspection service, but they cannot create administrative sanctions and, much less, invade the Union's sphere of competence.

In our opinion, this position adopted by Justice Cezar Peluso[92] is the most appropriate way to preserve and conserve water resources from the impacts that will undoubtedly be shared in the river basins now and in the future. This favours centralized planning that takes into account all the hydrographic basins and the shared hydro-environmental impacts and enables collective action (since it is the duty of the public authorities and society to preserve water resources) that is coherent and respects the unity of the watercourses. Centralized planning does not rule out decentralized action focused on common objectives, as it is possible to plan centrally and execute decentrally. This is what is proposed by Law 9.433/97, which extracted from this combination of competence rules a reading that makes centralized planning combined with decentralized action possible.

However, this is not what happens in practice in the states, which have a wealth of legislation that often clashes with federal legislation.

4.2. Material skills.

The material competences instrumentalized by the legislation produced by the

---

[92] STF: RE 194.704-MG.

respective federated entity make it possible to carry out the various activities entrusted to the Executive Branch[93] . In terms of water resources, the Union is exclusively responsible for establishing a national system for managing water resources and defining criteria for granting rights to their use (art. 21, XIX).

This competence only confirms the need for centralized legislation on water resources, with centralized planning and decentralized execution. In fact, the doctrine states that each "legislative competence corresponds to a specific administrative competence"[94] .

In proposing the creation of a national "system" for managing water resources, the constituent legislator recognized the need for uniform treatment of water resources, taking into account the geographical unity of the basin and the sharing of hydro-environmental impacts between water resources, reflecting the interconnection of all watercourses. Alongside this idea, it also introduced the need to coordinate and organize the actions of public authorities so that they function as an organized structure that respects this interrelated unity. Indeed, the term system includes the interconnection between the parts and the whole, as well as the coordinated interdependent relationship between the parts and the whole, which is why Vladimir Passos de Freitas states that

> The consideration of a system involves a whole character and in this recognition can help: a) identifying the relationship between the component parts; b) locating a pattern that governs the connections found; c) looking at the whole with the perception of a purpose[95] .

Thus, the mere mention of the adoption of a **system** to support the administrative protection of water indicates the recognition that there must be uniform treatment of all water

---

[93] "Under the Brazilian Constitution of 1967/69, administrative competence resulted directly and necessarily from the respective legislative competence. Therefore, an administration could not act to enforce the rules of another political sphere. On the other hand, no member state could, for example, prescribe to its municipalities the administrative procedure to be observed in their acts. According to the dominant theory in Brazil, such a regulation would abuse city halls, which would be reduced to 'bureaucratic intermediaries'". (KRELL, Andreas J. Discretion ..., p. 94).

[94] ANTUNES, Paulo de Bessa. Law ..., p. 75.

[95] FREITAS, Vladimir Passos de. Administrative Law ..., p.56.

resources in order to guide the components of the system in the same direction to achieve a common goal - preservation for present and future generations. Therefore, this constitutional orientation eliminates the possibility of subsystems legislating in their own cause to pursue a purpose other than that pursued by the central power of the system.

This uniform and inter-relational orientation that guides the establishment of the national system prevents the existence of a multiplicity of legal norms produced by the parts of the system (or subsystems) to define the purpose and common path to be pursued, since the subsystems only acquire an identity by fulfilling a macro function of the system.

The system's operative closure is instrumentalized by the centralization of legislative power in the federal sphere and its exclusive competence to create the national system, since otherwise we would have several systems (state and municipal, for example) chaotically producing countless objectives and thinking independently without seeking a common goal. This operational closure does not imply communicative closure with the environment and with the other systems.

It becomes possible, then, to use Luhmann's systemic theory - although it is not the aim of this work to analyze the entire National System in the light of this theory - to the extent that the constituent legislator, in having constitutionally idealized a national system for managing water resources, ends up conceiving a social system. This system is by definition autopoietic, i.e. "characterized by a self-reproducing and circular *perpetuum mobile* of acts of communication that generate new acts of communication"[96] .

In the systemic process there is a constant flow of communicative elements, which cause multiple effects and feed back into the system. All of this refers to the development and implementation of environmental policies, in other words, it is the system's own product, which we can generically consider as information for directing environmental actions and

---

[96] FARIAS, Paulo .ГсБё Leite. Water: economic or ecological legal asset? Brasilia: Brasilia Juridica, 2005, p. 298.

achieving the desired results[97] .

Heleno Taveira Torres includes the competence provided for in art. 23, XI of the CF/88 alongside the competence prescribed in art. 225, § 2 of the CF/88, as a competence aimed at guaranteeing the recovery of the degraded environment when exploiting said water resources. The author also points to the financial compensation prescribed in art. 20, § 1 of the CF/88 as an excellent environmental control instrument[98] .

4.3. Ownership of water resources.

The evolution of society towards recognizing environmental protection has diametrically affected the concept of the good. The starting point for these changes is the constitutional text itself, which, with a very progressive inspiration, even overcomes the position defended in 1978 at the Stockholm Convention by Brazilian representatives, according to which "Brazil was big enough to host all the polluting industries on the planet"[99] .

The starting point for any "patrimonial" analysis of the environment has to be art. 225 of the Federal Constitution, because, in addition to being a general provision of Environmental Law, it is also a provision that brings a holistic perspective to the environmental good[100] . The wording of the provision does not fragment the environmental good, but treats it as a whole, insofar as it considers that "everyone has the right to an ecologically balanced environment, which is a common use of the people and essential to the quality of life". There are no

---

[97] MILARE, Edis. Environmental law: doctrine, case law, glossary. 3. ed. rev., atual. e ampl., Sao Paulo: Editora Revista dos Tribunais, 2004, p. 393.
[98] TORRES, Heleno Taveira. The relationship ..., p. 108.
[99] VARELLA, Marcelo Dias. International Economic Law. Belo Horizonte: Del Rey, 2004, p. 30.
[100] CARVALHO, Edson Ferreira de. Meio ambiente & direitos humanos. Curitiba: Jurua, 2005, p. 323.

adjectives in this provision - such as gendic heritage, cultural heritage, artistic heritage etc. - which create micro-systems that are indifferent to shared impacts. As Leonard Boff says:

> Everything is related to everything at all points and at all times. No one lives outside this relationship. Even Darwin's law - that of the triumph of the strongest - is part of this pan-relationality and universal solidarity. It is because of the inter-relationships of all with all that diversity in all fields has been guaranteed, particularly biodiversity and the fact that we have all been able to reach the point we have today[101] .

The heading of art. 225 is also the starting point for their legal classification. The Constituent Assembly considered all environmental goods[102] - water, sea, soil, subsoil, fauna, flora, artistic, landscape, cultural - as goods of common use (art. 225) and as diffuse interests (art. 129, inc. III) and it is from this perspective that arts. 20 and 26 of the Republic's Charter should be read.

So one wonders: what kind of asset is environmental heritage? Is it public property or is it private property?

The first classification that comes to mind when we use the expression "goods for the common use of the people" is the one originally created in art. 66 of the Civil Code of 1916, and maintained by the Civil Code of 2002 in art. 99, in which public goods are classified: goods for the common use of the people, those for special use and dominical goods. It is with the 19th century view[103] that environmental goods tend to be classified as public goods[104] .

However, it should be borne in mind that this classification was created in a historical context in which the environment had, until recently, little or no importance *(res nullius* or

---

[101] BOFF, Leonardo. From the iceberg to Noah's Ark: the birth of a planetary ethic. Rio de Janeiro: Garramond, 2002, p. 98.

[102] There is no distinction between environmental resources and environmental goods.

[103] This vision was based on the principles of economic liberalism, which advocated a minimal state that did not interfere in private relations, guaranteed the right to property and preserved the autonomy of will.

[104] NUNES, Lydia Neves Bastos Telles. Property rights and water. *In:* A Tutela da agua e algumas implicacoes nos direitos fundamentals. Luiz Alberto David Araujo (Coord.), Bauru: ITE, 2002, p. 193.

coisa acessoria[106] [105]) for science, economics and law.

In the context of science, it should be remembered that Ren' Descartes maintained that all matter, with the exception of man who has a soul and consciousness, was governed by a mechanistic principle, so that it worked like a clock. Animals were mere machines, automated beings that didn't feel pain, which justified the atrocities committed against animals in the name of science.

Even Darwin's evolutionary theory, which could be read, in principle, as an awakening towards overcoming anthropocentrism - by placing man and animal on the same evolutionary line -, in reality, it more reflects the idea of the supremacy of man over all things and ends up influencing the Law in the sense of submitting the entire environment to the needs and well-being of man, regardless of a policy of preservation, which even appears today, in some sectors, as a form of self-preservation of the human species.

Economic policy was based on liberalism, which advocated minimal state intervention in relations between individuals and their property.

These relationships between science and economics and the law reflect the position adopted by the Civil Code of 1916, which classified goods as public (goods for the common use of the people, goods for special use and domain goods) and private. Environmental goods that were inexhaustible, and therefore did not need specific protection, were in fact considered *res nullius* or as accessory goods that would follow the fate of the principal (see the case of water where the

The owner of the land was usually the owner of the watercourses[106]). The 1916 Civil Code itself did not treat all environmental goods in the same way, in that some were considered to be public goods in common use owned by the State and others, such as fish in the water and loose poop, were *res nullius, owned by* those who conquered them.

---

[105] SILVA, Jos' Afonso da. Environmental Law..., p. 68.
[106] See articles 563 to 568 of the 1916 Civil Code and article 8 of the Water Code.

The same criticisms made of the concepts introduced by the 1916 Civil Code are perfectly applicable to the 2002 Civil Code, when interpreted without the Federal Constitution as the necessary starting point.

Today there are diffuse and collective interests, which go beyond the sphere of the private and even the public, pointing to a reflection on the old watertight dichotomy between public and private law, which is also reflected in the classification of public goods and private goods. This is a gray area in which the appropriation of environmental resources by the public authorities or private individuals is no longer admissible. This is because the government, despite its legitimacy to protect the environment, is, alongside private individuals, a powerful agent of degradation. For no other reason, the Public Prosecutor's Office has been given the task of defending diffuse interests.

In this regard, it is essential to point out that the recognition of diffuse interests is expressly based in Article 129, III of the Constitution. It should be noted that in this provision, the constituent legislator expressly introduces the figure of diffuse interests, which notably include the environment. It is therefore possible to conclude that the category of diffuse goods is constitutionally recognized.

Thus, by recognizing that there is no public or private ownership of environmental goods, the protection of environmental goods cannot be entrusted privately to the owner, to use the 19th century conception of the previous Civil Code, because, strictly speaking, everyone is an owner. For this very reason, the defense of the environment is attributed concurrently to citizens, through popular action; to the Public Authorities, through the exercise of police power, through public civil action - it should be noted that it is not possible to use petitionary actions in the defense of environmental goods; and to the Public Prosecutor's Office, through public civil action.

For this reason, Tc3ë Afonso da Silva, based on Italian doctrine, states that

According to Rui Carvalho Piva[108] , there seems to be no doubt in the legal profession as to the classification of environmental goods as diffuse goods. For him, the environmental good is undeniably a "diffuse good, a good protected by a right that aims to ensure a trans-individual interest, of an indivisible nature, owned by undetermined persons linked by circumstances of fact"[109] . The fact that it is a good in common use leads to the conclusion that there is no full ownership, bringing with it "the idea of collective legal bonds, diffuse as a species, which are established between undetermined people and goods in common use"[110] .

Under private law, the owner has the right to freely use, enjoy and dispose of the property. Environmental goods, which are of common use to the people and of diffuse interest by literal definition of the Constitution, cannot be subject to this regime. These are subject to their own legal regime.

Maria Sylvia Zanella di Pietro had already warned, with regard to common use and special use goods, that these goods were subject to

---

[107] SILVA, Afonso da. Environmental Law..., p. 83.
[108] PIVA, Rui Carvalho. Environmental Good. Sao Paulo: Max Limonad, 2000, p. 114.
[109] Ibid., p.114.
[110] Ibid, p.120.
[111] DI PIETRO, Maria Silvia Zanella. Private use of public property by private individuals. Sao Paulo: Editora

The legal regime to which environmental property is subject, in relation to private individuals and public authorities, is exclusively a legal regime of diffuse rights. This will have repercussions on the faculties attributed to "owners", which are to use, enjoy and dispose, "overlapping concepts"[112] . When ownership is full, all these faculties can be exercised, but when it is not, how do these faculties behave?[113] . It's true that the Constitution, by introducing the idea of the social function of property into the system, makes the exercise of these faculties conditional on their fulfillment, thus preventing them from being fully exercised. But it is also true that, in the case of environmental goods, these faculties are affected in their essence, being modified according to the good being protected. Let's take a look at each of these faculties.

The right to use, according to civilist doctrine, is one in which it is possible to "use the thing according to the owner's will and to exclude strangers from the same use"[114] or "the faculty to use is to put the thing at the service of the owner without altering its substance"[115] . However, with regard to diffuse goods, this system of private use by the government is not possible, which contradicts the idea of government ownership. In fact, as assets of diffuse ownership, the Government cannot absolutely prevent society from using them, but it can impose limitations that seek to preserve the environmental asset as much as possible. The elimination of any and all use by society goes against the diffuse nature of environmental goods. So much so that, even in fully protected conservation units, public visits are allowed for educational purposes (art. 9, §2, art. 10, §2, art. 11, §2, art. 12, §3 and art. 13, §3 of Law 9.985/2000).

The *jus fruendi* or right to enjoy, which can be confused in some cases with the right to use[116] , "involves the power to reap the natural and civil fruits of the thing, as well as to exploit

---

Revista dos Tribunais, 1983, p 5.

[112] PIVA, Rui Carvalho. Well..., p.122.

[113] No distinction is made between environmental goods and environmental resources.

[114] RODRIGUES, Silvio. Civil Law. 23. ed., Sao Paulo: Saraiva, 1996, v. 5, p. 74.

[115] VENOSA, Silvio de Salvo. Civil law: rights in rem. 2. ed., Sao Paulo: Atlas, 2002, p.159.

[116] DI PIETRO, Maria Silvia Zanella. Use ..., p. 5.

it economically, taking advantage of its products"[117] . In relation to this right of the owner, a distinguishing mark emerges between private property and "diffuse property". Environmental goods belong to everyone, but their economic exploitation can bring profit for some people (which is not shared by everyone) and shared social costs for all, which is why Garret Hardin[118] is concerned about them in his work "The Tragedy of the Commons". This is why, in the context of Environmental Economic Law, we advocate the internalization by economic agents of the negative externalities generated by production. It is with a view to minimizing these losses that environmental licensing, environmental zoning, environmental impact studies, environmental impact reports, among other instruments, are required, as well as why degraders are fined and ordered to restore the environment. In short, preventive and repressive measures are taken to control the enjoyment of environmental goods.

As you can see, in private law, the owner reaps the rewards, but is also responsible for the losses. In environmental law, this is not the case. Everyone who meets certain requirements can enjoy environmental goods, but the losses and social costs are always collective. Even if they are somehow internalized, it is society that will lose out, for example, with the extinction of a species of fauna or flora.

Public authorities and private individuals cannot alienate/dispose of a diffuse asset, not even if it were legally possible to do so - which, in the case of environmental assets, it is not - since the primary purpose of these assets is always to be preserved for present and future generations.

The concept of diffuse heritage does not fit into traditional legal models. In fact, this heritage includes assets of fundamental importance to life and the economy, such as water resources, so that the warning of Tc3ë is pertinent.

---

[117] RODRIGUES, Silvio. Law..., p. 74.
[118]
    HARDIN, Garret. The Tragedy of the Common Good. Translated by Prof. Tabajara Lucas de Almeida. Available at: http://www.dmat.furg.br/~taba/tragcomum.htm, Accessed on August 1, 2005.

Robson da Silva:

> Diffuse heritage includes goods that are necessary for life and the economy; goods that are at the frontier of the contemporary debate, such as geek heritage. These assets cannot be managed and guided only by the premises of dominance and the reasons of the state and private individuals. They must be guided by democratic access, the protection of human dignity and environmental protection. One of the critical problems in the area of assets that make up heritage, whether private, public or diffuse, is their management and access[119] .

Thus, the Government does not have *dominion over* environmental goods, but it does have the power to manage and police them[120] . With regard to goods in common and special use, as early as 1983, Maria Silvia Zanella Di Pietro stated: "to the faculties of use, enjoyment and availability, exercised in public law, in the manner indicated, are added the powers of management and policing that the Public Administration exercises over the goods it owns"[121] .

With this in mind, we bring together art. 20, inc. III and art. 26, inc. I of the Constitution of the Republic:

> Art. 20. The following are the property of the Union: (...) III - lakes, rivers and any streams of water on land under its control, or which border more than one state, serve as boundaries with other states, or extend to or from foreign territory, as well as marginal land and river beaches;
>
> Art. 26. The following are included among the property of the states: I - surface or subterranean waters, flowing, emerging and in deposit, except in this case, in accordance with the law, those resulting from Union works;

In these articles, public ownership of water is established, entrusted to the states and the Union. However, as we discussed above, environmental goods, including water, are not just public goods for the common use of the people, but also goods of diffuse interest. It has also been established that, as a result, the ownership of environmental goods in relation to the Government, in fact, is not such as to establish, in favor of the Union and the States, full

---

[119] SILVA, Jose Robson da. Paradigma ..., p. 279.
[120] MACHADO, Paulo Affonso Leme Machado. Brazilian Environmental Law. 11. ed., Sao Paulo: Malheiros, p. 423. SILVA, José Robson da. Op. cit., p. 285.
[121] DI PIETRO, Maria Silvia Zanella. Use ..., p. 6.

ownership, i.e. the *dominus of the* waters is not handed over, but only the management and policing power of this good.

By establishing the diffuse nature of water, it is possible to move on to the notion of managing water resources, introduced through the material competence described above (art. 21, XIX of the Constitution of the Republic). It follows that the public authorities and society will no longer be the owners of the asset, but the managers of water resources. Therefore, there is no other possible constitutional reading of articles 20, 26 and 225 of the Constitution, as far as the environmental good is concerned.

It follows that there will be three managers of the national water resources system - management, as we have seen, is decentralized, but governed by legislation centralized in the Union - namely: States, legitimized to join the system as members by virtue of Article 26, I, in order to privately manage the water resources mentioned therein; the Union, legitimized to privately manage the assets described in Article 20, III, VIII; and society, legitimized to manage all environmental assets by virtue of Article 225. This is the reason for the division of water resources between the States and the Union as assets "belonging" to these federal entities.

Management will be carried out through the system, created by the Union and, by virtue of its exclusive legislative power and the principle of predominance, it will also establish public water policies and define the institutes, principles and guidelines to be applied by the parts of the system. It is with these parameters in mind (private competence, exclusive material competence, diffuse ownership) that Law 9.4333/97 must be interpreted.

Chapter 5

Brazilian water resources management model.

5.1. National Policy and Management System.

The physical interdependence of water bodies[124] , the sharing of hydro-environmental impacts and the fundamental duty of the Government and the community to be jointly responsible for the preservation of environmental goods (art. 225, *caput, of* the CF/88) justify the choice of an integrated, participatory and decentralized management model for water resources.

In order to make this management model a reality, Law 9.433/97 established objectives, guidelines and instruments for the implementation of public policies for the preservation and conservation of water resources in the national territory, assigning the National Water Resources Management System the competence to implement this National Water Resources Policy (art. 32, inc. III, of Law 9.433/97).

It follows from this last competence (art. 32, inc. III) that the System, through its bodies, is determined to achieve the objectives of the National Policy, which are in summary:

---

[124] Normative Instruction of the Ministry of the Environment No. 4, of June 26, 2000, art. 2, item VI.

to ensure the availability of quantitatively and qualitatively adequate water for present and future generations (art. 2, inc. I); to promote the rational and integrated use of water (art. 2, inc. II) and to prevent and defend against critical hydrological events (art. 2, inc. III).[125]

Law 9.433/97 also talks about the specific objectives of the System, which are: to coordinate the integrated management of water (art. 32, inc. I); to arbitrate water conflicts (art. 32, inc. II); to plan, regulate and control the use, preservation and recovery (art. 32, inc. IV) and to promote water charges (inc. V). A systematic interpretation of the legal text reveals that the objectives set out in items I, II and IV of art. 32, strictly speaking, are means of guaranteeing the preservation of water resources, in order to ensure the availability of water and the rational and integrated use of water resources, i.e. they are means of implementing the objectives set out in art. 2. Item V, on the other hand, reveals an impropriety of legislative technique, since not only charging, but all the instruments must be implemented by the National System. Therefore, it can be seen that the only objective of the National System is, in fact, the implementation of the National Policy.

In order to enable coordinated action between the public authorities of the Union, the States and the Federal District, Law 9.433/97, in the exercise of private constitutional powers, outlines the scope of action of the State and District public authorities in the implementation of the National Policy. This is the meaning of Chapter VI of Law 9.433/97, which we will consider further below.

This chapter delimits the spheres of action of the state and federal executive powers, i.e. it distributes legal competencies in the matter of water resources, in order to integrate and coordinate the actions of the public powers. Thus, in implementing the National Policy, the state and district executive powers are responsible for: I - grant the rights to use water resources and regulate and supervise their use; II - carry out the technical control of water

---

supply works; III - set up and manage the Water Resources Information System, at state and Federal District level; IV - promote the integration of water resources management with environmental management. Note that the law allows the states and the Federal District to use two instruments: the grant (see also art. 14, §1) and the information system. This is because they have a closer perception of the water basins included in their territory.

5.2. Organizations and entities that make up the National System.

The National Water Resources Management System has as its component bodies (art. 33 of Law 9.433/97) the National Water Resources Council; the National Water Agency; the State and Federal District Water Resources Councils; the River Basin Committees; the federal, state, Federal District and municipal government bodies whose powers relate to water resources management; and the Water Agencies. Let's take a brief look at the function of each of these bodies, leaving the analysis of the Basin Committees for last, as it is the focus of this work.

The National Water Resources Council has the main functions of mediating water conflicts and articulating the integration of public policies on water resources, serving as a forum for debate and approval of national policy. It also has some normative functions, with regard to the matters in sections VI and X, when it establishes the criteria to guide national policy and for granting and charging (art. 35 of Law 9.433/97).[126] The State Councils function

---

[126] Law 12.334, of 2010, included three other sections: "XI - to ensure the implementation of the National Dam Safety Policy (PNSB); XII - to establish guidelines for the implementation of the PNSB, the application of its instruments and the operation of the National Dam Safety Information System (SNISB); XIII - to assess the Dam Safety Report, making recommendations, if necessary, to improve the safety of the works, as well as forwarding it to the National Congress."

similarly to the National Council.

The Water Agencies function as a technical body (the law allows each federal unit to opt for the legal model it will assume), where studies and surveys are carried out to support the drafting of national policy (art. 44 of Law 9.433/97).

The Basin Committees have their creation approved by an act of the National or State Water Resources Council and instituted by an act of the Chief Executive. Their area of action is the whole of a hydrographic basin or the sub-basin of a tributary of the main watercourse of the basin, or a tributary of that tributary or a group of contiguous hydrographic basins or sub-basins.

In these regions, the Committees will have the competencies established in Article 38 of Law 9.433/97[127] , among which the following deserve special mention, as they also emphasize the deliberative and decision-making nature of the body: to arbitrate, in the first administrative instance, conflicts related to water resources; to approve the basin's Water Resources Plan; and to establish the mechanisms for charging for the use of water resources and suggest the amounts to be charged.

The first of these competencies demonstrates a clear option for participatory democracy, insofar as it shifts the center of decision-making about conflicts from the ambit of the public administration alone to the ambit of a collegiate body with a plural composition, as will be seen below.

The second competence, highlighted in this work, demonstrates the intense popular

---

[127] Art. 38. It is the responsibility of the River Basin Committees, within the scope of their area of activity: I - promote the debate on issues related to water resources and coordinate the actions of the intervening entities; II - arbitrate, in the first administrative instance, conflicts related to water resources; III - approve the basin's Water Resources Plan; IV - monitor the implementation of the basin's Water Resources Plan and suggest the necessary measures to meet its targets; V - to propose to the National Council and the State Councils for Water Resources the accumulations, derivations, abstractions and connections of little expression, for the purpose of exemption from the obligation to grant rights to use water resources, in accordance with their domains; VI - establish the mechanisms for charging for the use of water resources and suggest the amounts to be charged; VII - (VETOED) VIII - (VETOED) IX - establish criteria and promote the apportionment of the cost of works of multiple use, of common or collective interest. Sole paragraph. The decisions of the River Basin Committees may be appealed to the National Council or to the State Water Resources Councils, according to their sphere of competence.

participation in defining the public policies to be pursued in the river basin, a true insertion of the citizen in the public space.

The third competency gives the Committee some control over the system, since the two main instruments of national policy, licensing and charging, are now directly influenced in their formulation by the body's plural decision.

The Committees are made up of representatives of the Union; of the States and the Federal District whose territories lie, even partially, in their respective areas of action; of the Municipalities situated, in whole or in part, in their area of action; of the water users in their area of action; of the civil entities for water resources with proven activity in the basin[128] .

In order to balance the power of community actors, Law 9.433/97 limited the representation of the executive powers of the Union, States, Federal District and Municipalities to half of the total number of members.

In addition, it should be noted that the Basin Committees function as a center of excellence for discussions, since the major local debates will be held within this body, marked by the presence of civil society and the state (art. 38 of Law 9.433/97).

5.3. Principles of the National Water Resources Policy.

By analyzing Law 9.433/97, it is possible to identify some principles that guide the National Policy and the application of its instruments: the principle of integrated and decentralized management; the principle of participatory management (or popular

---

[128] In the River Basin Committees of basins whose territories encompass indigenous lands, representatives of the National Indian Foundation (FUNAI) must be included, as part of the representation of the Union and of the indigenous communities residing there or with interests in the basin.

participation); the principle of multiple uses; the principle of the economic valuation of water; the principle of information; and the principle of sharing hydro-environmental impacts.

These norms are the guidelines of the National System, since management must always consider the entire hydrographic basin and be delegated to its multiple bodies to act within the scope of their competencies.

Water must be considered not only as a natural asset essential to life, but also as an asset with economic value. Thus, this standard allows us to recognize its value not only historically, but also as fundamental to the country's economic life.

The rule determining multiple uses conditions the application of the instruments, especially the grant, which must always, except in conditions of scarcity, allow the basin to be exploited to its full potential to serve as many purposes as possible.

Finally, the principle of participatory management or the principle of popular participation in water management shows that management must be committed to the realization of a radical democracy, since it allows society to participate in relevant decisions regarding water. It is a question of truly allowing citizenship to be built in the public space. Through the principle of participation, society is effectively allowed to influence relevant issues relating to water resources, since the law itself sets aside the old practice of handing administrative decisions solely to civil servants or committees. An example of this is the approval of the Basin Water Resources Plan, which establishes the desired uses for that water body (art. 38, inc. III of Law 9.433/97).

According to Tc3ë Robson da Silva:

> The state cannot be the sole manager of environmental goods, as these goods are part of society's diffuse heritage. This means that the management of public and diffuse assets cannot be considered democratic without popular participation. The management and control of water resources and geological resources, for example, must include the participation of the population. This will promote democratic access by the population to the benefits that economic exploitation can generate and, in addition, provide some control over both the definition of purposes and the use of

> th∋se resources. The conclusion is that control must be shared with civil society
> organized around a legal center, such as environmental, consumer and neighbourhood
> associations, etc.[129] .

In the system of Law 9.433/97, participation also takes place at the appellate level,
since the Basin Committees are part of the National Council. In fact, the Basin Committee is
the original venue for arbitrating conflicts. So, at least in theory, this law makes the principle
of participation a reality in every sense[130] .

The principle of information is present throughout Law 9.433/97, and it couldn't be
otherwise, since this principle is inextricably linked to the principle of participation. This is
because managing without information is fatally mismanaging. And popular participation
without information is legitimizing a dictatorship. The participation of the uninformed is a
maneuvering technique of the dominant power, in order to legitimize decisions under the
supposed guise of citizenship.

5.4. Instruments of the National Water Resources Policy.

The instruments are at the service of the National Policy and are intended to implement
its objectives, and each of the bodies and entities that make up the National System, in
accordance with centralized planning by the Union, will be entrusted with the task of
preserving, restoring and protecting water resources.

They are the following instruments: licensing, charging for the use of water resources,

---

[129] SILVA, Robson da. Paradigma ..., p. 276.

[130] "Participation should also take place in the administration's appeal bodies. These bodies act as a means of
getting the government to review its actions, without the need to go to court". (OLIVEIRA, Flavia de Paiva
Medeiros de. GUIMARAES, Flavio Romero. Law, Environment and Citizenship: an interdisciplinary approach.
Sao Paulo: Madras, 2004, p.107).

master plans, frameworks and the information system. These instruments have a close correlation, since the application of one often implies the use of information that is captured by the other as it is applied. Systemic functioning also comes into play here, since in order for the water resources management system to function effectively, "efficient communication between the subsystems and effective control mechanisms for their operation" must be established[131] . The instruments would be precisely these control mechanisms; and the subsystems, when applying the legislation, need to be in constant communication, retrieving the information from the communication.

The granting of the right to use water is one of the main instruments designed for the effective control of its operations, because it is through it that the Government will be able to maintain effective control of the quantity and quality of water in the river basin, making it possible to set targets to make the multiple uses compatible.

However, for the grant to be effective, the use must be compatible with the plan drawn up for the hydrographic basin (it is the plan that will determine which types of uses are compatible with the water body), respecting the framework of the water body[132] .

For example, a request for a permit to discharge effluents into a water body classified in the special class[133] , which is not compatible with receiving any type of emission, cannot be granted for use in the pulp industry (a use which involves discharging effluents), because it is recognized that the water body does not have the capacity to process this waste, as provided for in the Plan.

---

[131] FARIAS, Paulo Jose Leite. Water ..., p. 296.

[132] Resolution of the National Water Resources Council No. 12, of July 19, 2000.
Art. 2 The Water Agencies, within the scope of their area of operation, shall propose to the respective Hydrographic Basin Committees **the classification of bodies of water into classes according to their preponderant uses**, based on the respective water resources and environmental legislation and according to the procedures set out in this Resolution.

[133] CONAMA Resolution No. 357/2005. Art. 4 Fresh waters are classified as: I - special class: waters intended for: a) supply for human consumption, with disinfection; b) preservation of the natural balance of aquatic communities; and c) preservation of aquatic environments in fully protected conservation units. Art. 13: In special class waters, the natural conditions of the body of water must be maintained.

Granting is an instrument that is intertwined with charging, because only those uses that are not subject to it can be charged. The grant is always prior to the use. It can be preventive, which declares water availability in the Union's basins (art. 6 of Law 9.984/2000), or definitive, which allows the use itself from the outset.

Master plans are intended to support and guide the implementation of the National Water Resources Policy and the management of water resources and are drawn up[134] with a long-term planning horizon, in order to indicate the goals and solutions needed in the short, medium and long term.

The definition of the goals to be pursued and the local public policy guidelines for each river basin will be established through the master plans, taking into account the macro guidelines established in the national policy. The plans will be subsidized by the information collected by the water resources information system[135] . Law 9.433/97 sets out the minimum content of the plans, because, as it is a matter of setting public policies, an eminently administrative function, it is not possible to impose such legislative constraints as to prevent the system from being dynamic and adapting to reality, which is always in flux and changing.

According to Cid Tomanik Pompeu[136] , this should be in line with the planning of strategic sectors, such as the energy sector (National Electricity Plan[137]) and the shipping sector (National Travel Plan[138]). The author warns that

> The studies relating to the plans must be widely publicized and presented in the form of public consultations, convened by the River Basin Committee or, failing that, by the entity or management body. Society's participation in the stages of drawing up the

---

[134] The plans will be drawn up by the Water Agencies, supervised and approved by the Basin Committee, following the parameters set by law and observing the criteria indicated by the National Water Resources Council in Resolution 17 of May 29, 2001 (published in the Official Gazette on July 10, 2001).

[135] POMPEU, Cid Tomanik. Water law in Brazil. Sao Paulo: Editora Revista dos Tribunais, 2006, p. 234.

[136] Ibid, p. 235.

[137] Art. 1, sole paragraph of MME Ordinance 84, of April 17, 2000.

[138] Section 5 of Law 5.917, of September 10, 1973.

The National Water Resources Plan was approved by the National Water Resources Council Resolution No. 58 of January 30, 2006 (published in the Official Gazette on March 8, 2006), which addresses water resources with a holistic view of the country's hydrographic basins.

Framing is another instrument available for water management, as its purpose is to classify water bodies in order to adapt them to multiple uses. The framework, along with the grant[140] , are not recent instruments in Brazilian legislation: the latter dates back to the Water Code and the former was provided for in 1986 in Conama Resolution No. 20, June 18, 1986 (published in the Official Gazette on July 30, 1986).

Law 9.433/97, which inaugurated the Brazilian legal system, gave the national system the power to classify water bodies according to quality standards in order to establish specific parameters and indicators, with a view to making multiple uses compatible. The standard issued by CONAMA in 1986 continued to be adopted by the National System, even though it was not issued by one of its bodies. With a view to internalizing this standard in the system (through resonance), the National Water Resources Council issued Resolution No. 12 of July 19, 2000 (published in the Official Gazette of July 20, 2000), which formally incorporated the Conama Resolution into the National System as its own normative instrument.

However, on November 29, 2000, this time exceeding its remit, Conama issued a new Resolution, No. 274[141] , on the classification of water bodies, which partially revoked Resolution No. 20/1986. Years later, on March 17, 2005, Conama issued another Resolution,

---

[139] POMPEU, Cid Tomanik. op. cit., p. 235.
[140] Instrument provided for in the Water Code in art. 43, applicable to public waters.

[141] Published in the Official Gazette of January 8, 2001.

No. 357[142] , which totally revoked Conama Resolution No. 20/1986 and dealt with the classification of water bodies.

Although water is an environmental asset and CONAMA is the consultative and deliberative body of the National Environment System, the systemic complexity that determined the operational closure of the National Water Resources System ended up incorporating the standardization of the system's own mechanisms as a competence attributed to its structures. Therefore, the rules for framing water resources should be produced by the national water resources system itself and not by the national environment system, unless, by resonance, there is a structural coupling.

In any case, the framework is an important tool for helping in the decision-making process for preserving and conserving water resources.

The information system aims to collect information on the quantity and quality of water resources in each basin. This instrument acts as a unifying center for information on the various hydrographic basins. The information system avoids the dispersion and loss of information that is so essential to the implementation of the national water resources policy[143] .

Law 9.433/97 establishes that the entire structure of the system is obliged to provide information to the system (art. 25, sole paragraph). There can be no privileged or secret information in the system, in order to comply with the principles of popular participation and information.

Charging for the use of water resources, henceforth referred to simply as charging for water, will be discussed in greater depth in Chapter 7, but first it is necessary to outline some theoretical frameworks in the following chapter.

---

[142] Published in the Official Gazette of March 18, 2005.
[143] MACHADO, Paulo Affonso Leme. Resources ..., p. 89.

Chapter 6

Taxation in Environmental Law.

6.1 Taxation: a path to preservation? 6.1.1 Economic foundations: Arthur Pigou's theory and Pareto's Optimum theory. 6.1.2 Ethical foundations. 6.2. A question of fundamental law. 6.3. The polluter pays principle. 6.4. The extra-fiscal function of taxation. 6.5. Existential minimum immunity. 6.6. Taxation and water.

The subject of taxation in the context of environmental law is highly relevant, as taxation is a strong ally in the preservation and protection of the environment, and it can be used in its extrafiscal aspect both to discourage and stimulate behavior, through stricter taxation or the granting of tax incentives.

6.1. Taxation: a path to preservation?

There is no denying the fundamental importance of environmental preservation today, nor the imperative need to coordinate means and make efforts to give effect to the constitutional determinations on the duty of public authorities and society to preserve the environment and guarantee its maintenance for future generations, as called for in Article 225 of the Charter of the Republic. To this end, the state and society must find effective instruments to enable this conservation measure. Taxation is an alternative for achieving such a noble goal, given the difficulties involved in such an intertwining of principles and values[144][145]

.

Environmental taxation has a foundation, not just a legal one, which is supported by the polluter pays principle, extrafiscality and the theory of fundamental rights. The economic theories of Arthur Pigou and Pareto and the theory of an Earth ethic also point to taxation as a way of preserving the environment.

6.1.1. Economic foundation: Arthur Pigou's economic theory and Pareto's Optimum theory.

The theory of externalities was studied by Alfred Marshal in 1890 (in his work *"Public Goods and Externalities"*), but it was Arthur Cecil Pigou (1877-1959) who developed it in his book *"Economics of Welfare"*, later criticized by Ronald Coase in his work *"The problem of social cost"*[146] .

Arthur Pigou believed that the mere existence of externalities - which would be costs imposed or benefits given to people not taken into account in their actions - was enough to justify government intervention. He argued that if someone created a negative externality - such as pollution - then that person would become increasingly committed to the activity that

---

[144] TORRES, Heleno Taveira. The relationship ..., p. 97-98.

[145] SEBASTIAO, Simone Martins. Environmental Taxation. Curitiba: Jurua, 2006, p. 214.

[146] This article expanded the field of law and economics studies. Arthur Pigou's idea was that if an ox on my property destroyed my neighbor' s pasture, the government should intervene, preventing my cattle from grazing freely or at least imposing a heavy tax that would inhibit them from doing so, otherwise my cattle would continue to destroy my neighbor's pasture. For Ronald Coase, the solution to this problem would lie in a global system of property rights for private individuals, who would negotiate their interests, seeking an agreement in order to achieve an efficient internalization of external effects, with the State simply preventing the appearance of other externalities, in order to guarantee that internalization is complete. According to Richard Coase, the ideal would always be the prevention of externalities. (HENDERSON, David R. Biography of Ronald H. Coase. *In:* The Concise encyclopedia of economics. Available at: http://www.econlib.org/library/Enc/bios/Coase.html, retrieved on October 15, 2005 and SEBASTIAO, Simone Martins. Environmental Taxation. Curitiba: Jurua, 2006, p. 215).

generated the externality, and if someone created a positive externality - such as educating themselves and becoming a more interesting person to the world - they would never invest enough in education because they didn't realize the great importance of this act for society[147].

So, to discourage activity that caused a negative externality, Arthur Pigou advocated taxing that activity. To encourage activity that created a positive externality, according to him, the government should subsidize that activity. This is what economic theory calls Pigouvian taxes and subsidies[148].

Therefore, this author believes that the intervention of the state as a normative agent is fundamental for sustainable development, in the sense of normatively imposing the internalization of the costs of negative externalities through Pigouvian taxes. Thus, through state action, the impact of unbalanced economic exploitation is neutralized or reduced[149]. To the extent that the theory of correctness requires normative action (legal norms) by the state, taxation is legitimized as the most appropriate means of achieving a successful environmental policy.

Thus, for Arthur Pigou, there is an "optimal" level of pollution. The tax should be equivalent to the cost of the negative externality. The difficulty in obtaining the "optimum" rate lies in the measurement of environmental costs. Damage is measured in physical units such as tons of pollutants or concentration in the physical environment. On the other hand, there are synergy effects between various polluting sources, so estimating the economic value of a specific externality becomes a major obstacle. As there are major methodological difficulties in measuring and estimating the marginal costs of degradation, in practice the socially acceptable level of pollution is defined on the basis of criteria other than economic ones. This methodological difficulty is common to other public policies, such as the social

---

[147] HENDERSON, David R. Biography of Arthur Cecil Pigou (1877 - 1959). *In:* The Concise encyclopedia of economics. Available at: http://www.econlib.org/library/Enc/bios/Pigou.html, retrieved on October 15, 2005.
[148] HENDERSON, David R. Ibid.
[149] NUNES, Cleucio Santos. Tax law and the environment. Sao Paulo: DiaEtica. 2005, p. 135.

policy of health, education and even national security[150] .

As Cleucio Santos Nunes rightly points out:

> Pigou taxes are more efficient in achieving socio-economic optimum and are therefore preferred by economists. Comparing the adoption of environmental taxes with the regulation of permitted pollution rates, the effects on market equilibrium are barely perceptible and allocate high public resources. It should be noted that in order to monitor compliance with quotas for the release of effluents into a river or the air, for example, the state has to set up a technical and administrative structure which is usually expensive and whose maintenance costs will be passed on to society as a whole through general taxes on income, services and property.
> However, the great advantage of Pigou taxes is the extra-tax results. In a simple example, when the law determines that a factory will pay R$5,000.00 more in taxes on revenue than it earns from the sale of products resulting from a polluting industrial process, the industrialist's tendency will be to reduce or eliminate this cost from his product, since his competitor can manufacture the same or a similar good without this charge, and consumers will certainly opt to purchase the latter good. This rule, inherent to the market, forces the polluter to reduce production in order to pay less or to adopt techniques to clean up the environment they have polluted. This is much more convenient for socio-economic equilibrium than regulating pollution levels or quotas, because they accommodate the polluter. All they have to do is know that if they don't exceed the legal pollution levels, they won't suffer any extra costs on their products[151] .

But you can run into the situation where companies, through taxation, just pass on the cost to the employee in such a way as to produce social exclusion. To control this, the Pareto Optimum is perfectly in tune with environmental taxation. According to this idea (also called economic optimum), the product is a Pareto Optimum if, and only if, no agent or situation can be in a better position without causing another agent or situation to assume a worse position. Thus, "the tax must take into account the value of society's loss from pollution, and the monetary expression corresponds to the cost of cleaning up the property affected by the degradation. The tax, therefore, must take into account this repair cost in the same proportion or more"[152] . Cleucio Santos Nunes also warns:

> The application of a random calculation basis, based on an abstract value of the

---

[150]SOARES, Sebastiao Roberto. Environmental Management and Planning. Available at: http://www.ens.ufsc.br/~soares/aulaG2.pdf. Accessed on: July 9, 2005.
[151] NUNES, Cleucio Santos. Law ..., p. 135-136.
[152]NUNES, Cleucio Santos. Law ..., p. 140.

> environmental good, is difficult and tends not only not to inhibit the practice of
> polluting behavior - since it is easy to pass on the cost of the tax to the price of the
> product - but also does not help to change the attitude of the polluter in order to
> broaden their social view of the problem[153].

Environmental taxation, through the internalization of environmental costs, seeks to correct market distortions which, due to the dynamics of negative externalities, provide the polluting economic agent with a subsidy from society as a whole for the environmental costs it generates. The purpose of environmental taxation is to act as an instrument to induce economic agents (potential polluters) to behave in such a way that their actions are carried out in a way that is less costly to the environment. It is a mechanism for economic regulation and not for prohibiting/authorizing conduct[154].

6.1.2. Ethical foundation.

The ecological crisis is evident all the time. We are living at a time when the increasing destruction of nature is putting humanity itself at risk. It is estimated that between 1500 and 1850, one species was eliminated every ten years; between 1850 and 1950, one species per year; and from 1990 onwards, one species per day[155]. With this geometric escalation, in the next few decades one species should disappear every hour. There are also some clearly serious problems: desertification, whereby every year fertile land equivalent to the surface area of the state of Rio de Janeiro becomes desert; deforestation, whereby 42% of tropical forests have already been destroyed, and global warming combined with acid rain could decimate the 6 billion hectare boreal forest; overpopulation, which imposes an increasing demand on

---

[153] NUNES, Cleucio Santos. Law ..., p. 140.
[154] MODE, Fernando Magalhaes. Tributagao Ambiental, a função do tributo na protecção do meio ambiente. Curitiba: Jurua, 2003, pp. 112, 114 and 118.
   BOFF, Leonardo. Ecology: cry of the earth, cry of the poor. Rio de Janeiro: Sextante, 2004, p. 14.

environmental resources (note that in 1990 there were 5.2 billion people with a growth rate of between 3 and 4% per year, while food production increased by only 1.3%)[156] .

This crisis entered the debate of the international community in 1972, at the Stockholm Convention, where it became clear that the following paradigm had been broken for the first time: "that the world must revolve around the idea of progress. And that this progress moves between two infinities: the infinity of the Earth's resources and the infinity of the future. It was thought that the Earth's resources were inexhaustible and that we could progress indefinitely towards the future. The two infinites are illusory."[157] .

All this is a reflection of a humanist ethic that emphasizes human rights. "Ethics means doing good and avoiding evil, choosing the right and avoiding the wrong. The term right is at [155] the center of any ethic, and is used to protect certain values considered to be of fundamental [156] [157] importance to humanity."[158] .

Law has always been inspired by anthropocentric ethics, insofar as it should protect and regulate human behavior. Western philosophers justified "that only human beings are objects of moral concern and possess rights"[159] . It was with the ecological movement, despite the fact that it had existed and been systematized for a century and that ecologists were hardly heard[160] , that ideological, scientific, political, ethical and spiritual concerns now began to resonate in society and the international community.

> Ecology embodies an ethical concern, which is also demanded of all knowledge, powers and institutions: to what extent does each one collaborate in safeguarding threatened nature? To what extent does each area of knowledge incorporate the ecological, not as an additional theme in its research, leaving its specific methodology unquestioned, but to what extent does each area of knowledge redefine itself based on the ecological question and thus become a homeostatic factor, that is to say, a factor of ecological balance, dynamic and creative. Rather than disposing of reality as he pleases or mastering dimensions of nature, human beings must learn how

---

Ibid., p. 16.
Ibid., p. 15.
[158] CARVALHO, Edson Ferreira de. Meio ambiente & direitos humanos. Curitiba: Jurua, 2005, p. 321.
[159] Ibid, p. 322.
[160] BOFF, Leonardo. Ecology ..., p. 16.

to manage or deal with nature by obeying the logic of nature itself or, starting from within it, enhance what is already found within it. Always with a view to its preservation and further development[161].

From this ecological perspective, which states that no element or activity should be considered in isolation, due to the circularity and holistic basis of ecosystems[162] , Aldo Leopold argued in his work "Earth Ethics" (1949) that not only human beings, but also plants, animals and nature have rights, rejecting the image of man as dominator of the earth[163] . Aldo Leopold formulated the concept of the biotic community, which is the

> The translation of a scientific reality (ecological holism), the object of a shared love which is itself the fruit of a long historical maturation of ethics, the 'biotic community' is the culmination of a new ethic. It enshrines, of course, the right to existence and the natural development of each of its elements and, consequently, changes the role of *Homo sapiens:* from being a conqueror of the earthly community, he is called to become its full-time member[164] .

A new paradigm is being introduced in law, for some the biocentric, and for others the holistic, through which the atomistic approach to rights is abandoned for holistic and systems processes. With biocentrism, the legal system promotes and recognizes rights for the biotic and abiotic environment[165] , and the concept of heritage takes on new meanings[166] .

> In this respect, Aldo Leopold launched the moral criterion for evaluating the rightness or wrongness of human behavior in relation to the environment by stating that 'we can judge our relationship with the non-human world as right when it tends to preserve the integrity, stability and beauty of the biotic community and as wrong when it tends in the opposite direction'[167] .

---

[161] Ibid., p. 18.

[162] The idea of an interconnected whole was developed by the Gaia theory, based on the idea that the Earth is a living organism in which everything is intimately connected.

[163] CARVALHO, Edson Ferreira de. op.cit., p. 322.

[164] Aldo Leopold *apud* OST, Frangois. Nature outside the law - ecology in the face of the law. Translated by Joana Chaves. Lisbon: Institute Piaget, 1995, p. 190.

[165] See also Christopher Stone ("Should trees have standing?"), where the author proposes the extension of rights to forests, rivers and other natural objects. Also in a similar vein is James Nash with his theory of biotic rights ("The case for biotic rights").

[166] SILVA, Jose Robson da. Paradigma ..., p.369.

[167] CARVALHO, Edson Ferreira de. Meio ..., p. 323.

For Jose Robson da Silva, this paradigmatic shift is evident in our Constitution in art. 225, item VII, of the CF/88, which prohibits, in the form of the law, practices that jeopardize their ecological function, cause the extinction of species or subject animals to cruelty, conferring, in the author's view, the right to flora and fauna, giving them the quality of subjects of rights[168] .

At the international level, to a certain extent, the paradigmatic shift can be seen "in international environmental regulation, which has included the ecosystem in its range of issues, such as the Biodiversity Convention"[169] .

Along these lines of an ecological moralist movement[170] , Michel Serres proposes the natural contract. For him, nature behaves like a subject of law[171] . For this reason, man must revalue it as an equal in order to negotiate and conclude a natural contract (along the lines of the social contract).

Michel Serres explains that it would be like a return to classical natural law, with the addition of globality and symbiosis[172] . In order to ensure the will of nature, Michel Serres proposes two ways: to invoke the purely tacit and virtual nature of the natural contract, since as in the social contract it remains unsigned and operative, being a condition for the possibility of the natural state[173] of cohabitation with nature[174] ; or to understand, as he seems to prefer, that

---

[168] SILVA, Jose Robson da. op. cit., p.208.

[169] CARVALHO, Edson Ferreira de. Meio ..., p. 324.

[170] STO, Frangois. Nature on the fringes of the law - ecology at the mercy of the law. Translated by Joana Chaves. Lisbon: Instituto Piaget, 1995, p. 189.

[171] "Qu'est-ce que la nature? D'abord l'ensemble les conditions de la nature humaine elle-meme, ses contraintes globales de renaissance ou d'extinction, l'hotel qui lui donne logement, chauffage et table; de plus elle les lui ote des qu'il en abuse. It conditions his tour. La nature se conduit comme un sujet". (SERRES, Michel. Le contrat naturel. Paris: Flamarion, 1992, p. 64.)

[172] "Since then, men have returned to the world, the world to the global, the collective to the physical, a little like at the time of classical natural law, but with great differences, qui tiennent toutes au passage recent du local au global et au rapport renouvele que nous entretenons desormais avec le monde, notre maitre jadis et naguere notre esclave, toujours notre hote en tous cas, maintenant notre symbiote". (Ibid, p. 67.)

[173] "We are there," Kant would have said, "in the transcendental order: the social contract would be the condition for the possibility of the civil state (...)" (OST, Frangois. op. cit., p. 195.).

[174] SERRES, Michel. op. cit., p. 69 and 78.

"the Earth speaks to us in terms of forces, bonds and interactions, and this is enough to make a contract"[175] .

Josd Robson da Silva seems to be moving in this direction when he states that, "going beyond the philosophy of ownership, an environmental code can be guided by a natural contract in which the person is not separated from nature, but, on the contrary, is recognized in it because the contract that man has made with nature is recent and the protection of all life is a paradigm that is being installed at the constitutional level"[176] .

For Francois Ost, the most favorable reading of Michel Serres would be the third part of his work (Science, Law[177]), which highlights the following:

> The real question that Michel Serres' work raises from the outset, albeit in filigree, on the subject of the natural contract, is that of the government of men by science; or, better still, the necessary confrontation between legal guarantees (prudence, contract, justice, balance of services) and scientific knowledge. The legal system has so far managed to pacify relations between men; this is the role of the social contract. Science, on the other hand, has never lost the world; the wise contract or scientific contract on which it is based "gives the reason" for things in the world. The question today is to overlap the two contracts: to reintegrate the interest of the world into the commerce of men.
> (...) Reducing the natural contract to a critical collaboration between the politician who decides and the scientist who informs, this is surely the most favorable reading that can be made of Michel Serres' work, on the condition that we don't fall into the scientism (government by science) that we often fall into[178] .

As you can see, there is a concrete and significant effort to recognize the intrinsic value of the environment, with the only difference being how this is done. While "some argue that this recognition can be done in the context of legal rights, others argue for the recognition of nature's values, which should be taken into account by humanity when establishing its priorities"[179] .

It would be naïve not to recognize that such a profound paradigmatic shift is free from

---

[175] Ibid., p. 69.
[176] SILVA, Jose Robson da. Paradigma ..., p.245.
[77] SERRES, Michel. The contract..., p. 87-140.
[178] STO, Francois. Nature...., p. 196.
[179] CARVALHO, Edson Ferreira de. Meio ..., p. 328.

criticism. In practice, many people do not find ways to grant innate rights to the environment without giving it a means of defense. On the other hand, implementing this paradigm while ignoring the anthropocentric tradition of the sciences, especially law, which finds its great core in fundamental rights, is unlikely, because "paradoxically, biocentric ethics is anthropocentric in that it would be impossible to imagine the existence of any system of values independent of human beings, who are the only ones capable of making value judgments"[180] .

As Francois Ost explains,

> Law is a cultural product, it emanates from the ideas, fears and desires of men, and the reference to nature does not alter this fact in any way, except insofar as it offers more variety (not the least seductive, however) of the inexhaustible arguments that people invent in order to believe and be believed.
> But if it is for men, law is also for men, and for this simple but inescapable reason, the language it speaks has no meaning except for them (...)
> One of the fundamental theses of this work is to maintain that the concern that is beginning to emerge today, in political discourse and legal texts, for the future hosts of the planet - that is to say, the attention paid to future generations - should make it possible to ensure a disinterested and long-term protection of the environment, while at the same time not rejecting the framework, which we believe to be insurmountable, of practical humanism (...)....] Ecosphere protection and concern for future generations are dialectically linked. At the same time, we will have preserved the framework of legal humanism while extending it to the men and women of tomorrow: this, it seems to us, is the only real historical continuity (so often invoked by *deep ecologists) that is* needed. Moving from love for oneself to love for one's neighbor, and from one's neighbor to the far-off. To take the universalization inherent in the ideal of human rights to the extreme limits of time and space.[181]

Along these lines comes Jose Rubens Morato Leite, who defends the broadening of the anthropocentric paradigm to provide a repersonalization of the Law, through the perception that the Law makes sense when it is structured and functionalized around the rights of the human person and that the human person is responsible for nature, and therefore assumes the position of guardian of the biosphere. This re-personalization extends classical anthropocentrism and incorporates concerns about the environment and gives rise to "a solidarity of interest between man and the biotic community of which he is an interdependent

---

[180] CARVALHO, Edson Ferreira de. Meio ..., p. 328.
[181] STO, Francois. Nature...., p.215.

and integral part. It can be seen that responsibility for the integrity of nature is a condition for ensuring man's future"[182] .

We believe that extending anthropocentrism to include the protection of nature with a view to protecting future generations is the best way forward. Indeed, biocentrism, despite its noble direction, seeking to warn and break with a devastating culture, is much more of a symbolic strategy that we don't know for sure if it will bring results. We agree with Frangois Ost's warning:

> But symbolism, in law as elsewhere, is a delicately handled mixture. It could well work in reverse to the expected effect or generate perverse effects. In this case, the risk that the abuse of the reference to fundamental rights and the proliferation of pseudo-subjects will ultimately lead to a loss of credibility on both sides is, we believe, real[183] .

However, we believe that the important thing is to recognize that the world is in danger and that we have to rethink the way we treat nature. Law must internalize a new ethic, either by incorporating values into anthropocentrism that make it possible to protect nature, or by changing the paradigm. What is certain is that these reflections are felt in the law, which increasingly justifies action not only by the government but also by the community in general, using all means to achieve environmental preservation. From the above, it can be seen that if environmental taxation is a suitable means of achieving the protection of nature, then it should be implemented.

6.2. A question of fundamental rights.

The economic and philosophical approach to the environment presents instruments that

---

[182] LEITE, Jose Rubens Morato. Dano ambiental: do individual ao coletivo, exptrapatrimonial. 2. ed. rev., atual. e ampl., Sao Paulo: Editora Revista dos Tribunais, 203, p. 75.
[183] STO, Frangois. Nature...., p.215.

legitimize environmental taxation as a way of preserving the environment. Alongside these arguments, it is impossible not to mention the support of the theory of fundamental rights for instituting environmental taxes. Therefore, the theory of fundamental rights emerges as a central argument in the study of the problem in question, in which arguments are sought to legitimize environmental taxation in the field of water resources.

It is not possible to pretend that the rules that prescribe fundamental rights are only extracted from the normative statements contained in the Constitution. Pontes de Miranda warns that "it would be a mistake to believe that the mere fact that a reference to a right is included in the Constitution, and therefore does not allow it to be altered by ordinary law, makes it fundamental" [184]

Fundamental law norms are characterized by structural openness[185] . However, this does not mean that every rule can be classified as a rule of fundamental law. According to Robert Alexy, the norms extracted from the statement must maintain a relationship of precision and/or a relationship of foundation.

The *relationship of precision is* present when the norm expressed in the constitutional text (enunciation) is applied in concrete cases, in other words, it is a specification of a manifestly open provision. Thus, an unwritten fundamental right is not in a relationship of precision, but of justification.

As the text of the Constitution contains the **precise norm**[186] - a logical consequence of the enshrinement of a certain fundamental right - this type of norm becomes a *sine qua non* for the existence of the **norm that must be precise**. It is between the two norms that the

---

[184] MIRANDA, Pontes de. Comentarios a Constituigao de 1967. Sao Paulo: Editora Revista dos Tribunais, 1967, t. IV, p. 621.
[185] ALEXY, Robert. Teoria de los Derechos Fundamentales. Madrid: Centro de Estudios Constitucionales, 2002, p. 68.
[186] In the original: "norma hay que precisar y la norma precisante". (ALEXY, Robert. Teoria de los Derechos ..., p. 70).

relationship of foundation is established[187] .

Through these relationships, it is justified to conceive as fundamental right norms not only the norms explicitly stated directly in the constitutional text but also those that derive from its provisions[188] , similar to what art. 5, §2 of the Federal Constitution establishes. These resulting norms would be what Alexy calls "adscripted norms".

Fundamental law norms can thus be divided into two groups: 1) fundamental law norms directly laid down by the Constitution; and 2) fundamental law norms that derive from the Constitution (which Robert Alexy calls "adscripted norms")[189] . The latter will be fundamental law norms if the jusfundamental argument[190] can justify them as a possible

---

[187]In other words: The relationship of foundation occurs between the norm that must be specified and the precise norm, because the latter (the norm that must be specified) must exist since the text of the Constitution contains the former (the precise norm), which would be a logical consequence of the enshrinement of a certain fundamental right.

[188] In the original: "conceir como normas de derecho fundamental no solo las normas que son expresadas directamente a travds de enunciados de la Constitution, sino tambidn las normas del tipo presentado" (ALEXY, Robert. op. cit., p. 70).

[189] Alexy teaches that "an inscribed norm is worthwhile and is a fundamental law norm if it is possible to give a correct iusfundamental reasoning for its inscription in a directly established fundamental law norm". He further informs that: "normas de derecho fundamental pueden, por ello dividirse em dos grupos: em las normas de derecho fundamental directamente estatuidas por la Constitution y las normas de derecho fundamental a ellas adscriptas". (Ibid., p. 70).

[190] To complete the concept of an "encrypted norm", Robert Alexy uses his theory of legal argumentation, in which he states that this (legal argumentation) is a special case of general practical discourse (Habermas). According to this logic of rational reasoning, the specific rules of legal discourse are applied, while the general rules of practical discourse are also used when they are insufficient. For him, legal discourse means that: **1)** in legal discourse, practical issues are discussed; **2)** there is a claim to correctness; **3)** in legal discourse, propositions are intended to be rational within the framework of the legal system in force (it is not intended to judge which proposition is the most rational). Legal discourse has specific rules and forms, such as that propositions must be subject to the law, judicial precedents and dogmatics. He emphasizes two aspects in the justification of legal decisions: internal justification (validity of the inference) and external justification (conformity of the premises). He formulates the following rules for legal discourse: 1) The first two rules of internal justification must be satisfied: a) In order to justify a legal decision, at least one universal norm must be presented. b) The legal decision must be logically followed by at least one universal norm, together with other propositions. 2) Every form of argument that should be included among the canons of interpretation must be saturated. 3) Arguments that express a connection with the literal content of the law or with the will of the historical legislator prevail over others, unless other rational reasons can be presented that give priority to other arguments. 4) The weight of different arguments must be determined according to weighting rules. 5) Consideration should be given to all the arguments that can be put forward, and that can be included, by their form, among the canons of interpretation. The following rules apply to argumentation in the context of dogmatics: 1) If in doubt, every dogmatic statement must be substantiated by at least one general practical argument. 2) Every dogmatic statement must be able to be systematically proven, in both the strict and broad sense. 3) If dogmatic arguments are possible, they must be used. As rules for the use of precedents, Alexy lists the following: 1) When it is possible to cite a precedent for or against a decision, this should be done. 2) Whoever wishes to depart from a precedent assumes the burden of the argument. For the use of special legal arguments, Alexy formulates the following rule: the forms of special legal arguments must be saturated. (ALEXY, Robert. Legal Argumentation Theory: the theory of rational discourse as a theory of legal reasoning. Translation by Zilda Hutchinson Schild Silva; technical revision of the translation and

judgment .[191]

Within the current constitutional scheme, which underpins the jusfundamentality of a right, a catalog of fundamental rights and guarantees can be found directly in Title II of the Federal Constitution, i.e. this Title points to fundamental right norms directly laid down by the Constitution. This catalog, however, is opened up by §2 of art. 5 of the Charter of the Republic[191 192].

For Përe/ Luno, who adopts the term "derechos humanos"[193], instead of fundamental rights[194], they are a set of faculties and institutions which, at each historical moment, make concrete the demands of human dignity, freedom and equality, which must be positively recognized by legal systems at national level[195].

Taking the theory of fundamental rights (Robert Alexy and Perez Luno) as a starting point, the doctrine has uniformly understood - despite the fact that it is not expressly included in art. 5 of the Constitution of the Republic, which strictly speaking, as seen in Robert Alexy, is not a prerequisite for it to be considered a fundamental right - that the right to an ecologically balanced environment is a fundamental right. It cannot be denied that its content is that of a fundamental right, and it can even be said that the precepts of art. 225 of the Federal Constitution enshrine an environmental policy and a legal duty for the Government to preserve it[196]. In the words of Edis Milare:

> In addition to the individual and collective rights and duties listed in Article 5, the constituent legislator added a new fundamental right of the human person in the

---

introduction to the Brazilian edition by Claudia Toledo. 2. ed., Sao Paulo: Landy Editora, 2005, p. 210 and following).

[191] "Whether or not an inscribed norm is a fundamental right norm depends on the iusfundamental argumentation that is possible for it." (ALEXY, Robert. Teoria de los Derechos ..., p. 71).

[192] Fundamental rights can also be found in the international order, in treaties, including, in our opinion, in the Fundamental Declarations, as they contain universal human rights.

[193] LUNO, Antonio E. Perez. Fundamental Rights. Madrid: Tecnos, 2004, p.46.

[194] Insofar as we adopt a broad anthropocentrism, the term human rights identifies with this option, although we prefer the term fundamental rights due to its more universal and widespread nature.

[195] LUNO, Antonio E. Perez. op. cit., p.46.

[196] LEITE, Jose Rubens Morato. Damage..., p. 87.

caput of Article 225, aimed at the enjoyment of adequate living conditions in a healthy environment or, in the words of the law, "ecologically balanced"[197] .

For Jose Rubens Morato Leite, this qualification as a fundamental right results in a dual legal nature, being both a subjective right of the personality of a public nature and a fundamental element of the objective order[198] . The author explains:

> It is a subjective right of the personality in the sense that it is possible for all individuals to claim the right of defense against acts harmful to the environment, since its ecologically balanced preservation is a condition for the development of the human personality. This subjective right to defend the environment, which is public in nature, can be exercised on an individual basis (art. 5, item LXXIII, of the 1988 Constitution), not in relation to an exclusively individual interest, but in relation to a collective or diffuse environmental interest. Rota, emphasizing the subjective nature of the right to an ecologically balanced environment, says that it belongs to each and every human being, without its collective exercise conditioning its instruments of protection at the legal level. It is a subjective right with a solidarity profile, i.e. not a selfish profile, but rather, according to Pureza, a right-function.
>
> The objective dimension of the environment, i.e. its second nature, is immediately apparent in § 1 of art. 225 of the Federal Constitution, when the State is entrusted with essential tasks in environmental preservation. As we have already seen, these are unavoidable duties of the Environmental Law State, with a view to achieving environmental equity.
>
> Sendim, when dealing with the subject, reinforces this point of view, stressing that the objective dimension is ensured by the constitutionally stipulated norms of purpose and norms of task, which require the powers that be and, in the first place, the legislator, to protect and promote them.

Celso Antonio Pacheco Fioriolo qualifies them as diffuse rights[199] , escaping the classic dichotomy of public and private, since they would not be attributed to private individuals or to the State, but to "everyone" and to the "State", in the words of art. 225 of the Federal Constitution[200] . They would be rights marked by the degree of importance for the survival of this and future generations .[201]

---

[197] MILARE, Edis. Law ..., p. 137.
[198] LEITE, Jose Rubens Morato. op. cit., p. 88.
[199] It is important to note that the aforementioned author also qualifies the right to an ecologically balanced environment as a fundamental right.
[200] FIORILO, Celso Antonio Pacheco. Course in Brazilian environmental law. 4. ed., Sao Paulo: Saraiva, 2003, p. 5.
[201] SILVA, Jose Robson da. Paradigma ..., p. 273.

The Federal Supreme Court recognizes that the right to an ecologically balanced environment is a fundamental right, as can be seen in the following sentence:

> [...] The question of the right to an ecologically balanced environment - third generation right - principle of solidarity. - The right to the integrity of the environment - a typical third-generation right - constitutes a legal prerogative of collective ownership, reflecting, within the process of affirmation of human rights, the significant expression of a power attributed, not to the individual identified in his singularity, but, in a truly broader sense, to the social collectivity itself. [...] (STF - MS 22.164 - SP - T.P. - Rel. Min. Celso de Mello - DJU 17.11.1995)

Therefore, based on the rules of legal discourse, which underpin Alexy's definition of a fundamental right, it can be seen that the constitutional norm of art. 5, § 2, as well as the doctrinal concepts of Perez Luno, Jose Rubens Morato Leite, Paulo Afonso Leme Machado and Edis Milare, as well as the long-standing case law, confer the "status" of a fundamental right on the right to an ecologically balanced environment.

From this perspective, laшбёш the right of access to water resources (an environmental asset) that are quantitatively and qualitatively appropriate for their multiple uses (prioritizing human consumption and animal watering) takes on the legal nature of a fundamental right[202] . Thus, the right of access to water can be understood as a fundamental right of the human person, given that without this environmental resource, the existence of life is denied.

> The existence of human beings - in itself - guarantees them the right to consume water and air: 'Water is the right to life'. Therefore, it is correct to say that denying human beings water is denying them the right to life; in other words, it is condemning them to death. The right to life is prior to other rights. 'The relationship that exists between man and water precedes the law. It is an intrinsic element of their survival'[203]

---

[202] Stockholm Declaration of 1972. Principle 2 - The Earth's natural resources, including air, water, soil, flora and fauna, and especially representative parts of natural ecosystems, should be conserved for the benefit of present and future generations through careful planning or appropriate management. Available at: http://www.silex.com.br/leis/normas/estocolmo.htm

[203] MACHADO, Paulo Affonso Leme. Resources ..., p. 13-14.

It must be emphasized that, as long as the environmental asset is sufficient to fulfill the priority task of serving human consumption and, subsequently, animal watering, it must meet other uses. In this sense, Paulo Afonso Leme Machado teaches: "Public authorities are explicitly forbidden from granting rights of use that only allow for a single use of water."[204] We disagree, in part, with what the author says, insofar as water can have a single use (human consumption) when this resource is not quantitatively sufficient for other uses.

According to this broad doctrinal explanation, there is no denying that there is a fundamental right to a healthy environment. This recognition leads to a second affirmation, in the sense that there is a fundamental right of access to the environmental good (water) in sufficient quantity and quality to protect the vital minimum and the ecological minimum.

So how can it be conceived that Law 9.433/97 prevents free access to water for everyone who needs it? To answer this question, it is first necessary to review the theories that explain how to proceed with restrictions on a fundamental right.

There are two theories that try to explain the restrictions on fundamental rights: the external theory and the internal theory.

The external theory conceives that there is a difference between the right and its restrictions, separated by a special relationship, namely that of restriction. Once this relationship is accepted, then it can be concluded that there is "firstly, the right itself, which is not restricted, and secondly, what is left of the right when the restrictions are removed, that is, the restricted right"[205] . For this theory, there is no necessary relationship between the concept of right and that of restriction. There would only be a (non-necessary) relationship forged as a result of a need external to the law, which needs to find ways to reconcile the rights of

---

[204] Ibid., p. 34.
[205] ALEXY, Robert. Theory of Rights..., p. 268

different individuals, in their individual and collective aspects, as well as collective goods[206] . This theory is closely linked to the individualist conception of the state and society.

The internal theory does not distinguish between rights and restrictions, for it what exists is a right of a certain content. The concept of restriction is replaced by that of limit. Thus, this theory seeks to define the content of the right. In this way, "immanent restrictions" are recognized in the right[207] . This theory portrays the assumption of the individual as a member of a community.

Robert Alexy explains that

> The correctness of the external or internal theory depends, essentially, on whether the iusfundamental norms are considered as rules or principles and the iusfundamental positions as definitive or *prima facie positions*. If from definitive positions, it is possible to refute the external theory; if from *prima facie* positions, the internal theory.

Thus, depending on the starting point in the specific case, we may or may not be talking about restrictions on fundamental rights.

Once the restrictions on fundamental rights are theoretically situated, we move on to define them. Restrictive are the goods that are protected by the law (freedoms / situations / positions of ordinary law) and the *prima facie* positions granted by the principles of the law[208] .

The goods protected by the jusfundamental principles require broad protection. Therefore, a restriction on these goods will always be a restriction on a "prima facie" position granted by the fundamental right principle. Hence Alexy's preliminary assertion that "therefore, to the question of what restrictions on fundamental rights are, a simple answer is offered: restrictions on fundamental rights are norms that restrict prima *facie* iusfundamental

---

[206] Ibid., p. 268
[207] Ibid., p. 269.
ALEXY, Robert. Teoria de los Derechos ..., p. 272.

positions*"209*.

It should be noted that a rule restricting a fundamental right must be compatible with the constitutional text or the constitutionality bloc[210] , i.e. it must be constitutional, otherwise it would be a real undue intervention in the subject's sphere of freedom. Thus, the characteristic of rules that restrict fundamental rights is their compatibility with the constitutional text.

Alexy offers the following concept:

> Here we will present one that, but only of the norms restricting mandate and prohibition, refers to all regressive norms: the restrictions of fundamental rights are norms that restrict the realization of iusfundamental principles[211] .

Alexy points to two types of restrictions on fundamental rights: directly constitutional restrictions and indirectly constitutional restrictions.

Directly constitutional restrictions are made through a rule of constitutional stature, while indirectly constitutional restrictions are promoted by rules hierarchically inferior to the Constitution, which are authorized by the latter to make such restrictions[212] .

In order to understand restrictions, a distinction must be made between a restriction and a restrictive clause.

> The concept of restriction corresponds to the perspective of the right; that of a restrictive clause, to the perspective of the norm. Una clausula restrictiva es la parte de la norma completa de derecho fundamental que dice como esta restringido o puede ser restringido lo que el supuesto de hecho fundamental garantiza *prima facie*[213] .

We will now take a closer look at the indirectly constitutional restrictions, as they are essential for solving the proposed problem, which is to define the legal nature of water charges.

Ibid., p. 272.
In Brazil, the constitutional bloc includes, in addition to the constitutional text, treaties and customs.
[211] ALEXY, Robert. Teoria de los Derechos ..., p. 276.
[212] Ibid., p. 277.
[213] Ibid., p. 277.

As defined above, indirectly constitutional restrictions are those whose imposition is authorized by the Constitution. The power to impose directly constitutional restrictions is contained in the reserve clauses.

Explicit reservation clauses are those jusfundamental provisions or parts of jusfundamental provisions that expressly authorize interventions, restrictions or limitations.

There are powers to impose restrictions not only where the Constitution expressly determines them, but also in implicit reserve clauses. "Every time ordinary laws are referred to as restrictions, a power to impose restrictions is established"[214] .

The Constitution, by recognizing the need to manage water resources and establishing criteria for granting them, implicitly determines that the unlimited and disorderly use of this environmental asset should be restricted by law, in order to preserve it quantitatively and qualitatively for present and future generations.

In this sense, Fabiana Santos Dantas states that

> Management is of fundamental importance to its preservation, because only through rational and systematic management is it possible to produce, distribute and regulate the demand for and use of water resources, guaranteeing fair and equitable access for all[215] .

Thus, the notion of management brings with it the idea of the rational use of water, in other words, it opens up the possibility of restricting the use of water through criteria to be established legally. The very reference to the grant in the constitutional text serves as an indication that there will be control over use, since the primary objective of this instrument is to regulate it, setting quotas for derivations and abstractions in order to maintain quality

---

[214] ALEXY, Robert. Teoria de los Derechos ..., p. 283.
[215] DANTAS, Fabiana Santos. Water Resources Management: a critical analysis of Law 9.433/97. *In:* The application of environmental law in the federal state. Adreas J. Krell (org.) Rio de Janeiro: Editora Lumens Juris, 2005, p. 267.

standards.

It is clear that Law 9.433/97 functions as an indirectly constitutional restrictive rule. Thus, if the right to use water, as seen above, is a fundamental right and if management, to be established by law in accordance with the provisions of articles 21, inc. XIX and 23, inc. IV of the Federal Constitution, is a way of restricting this right, then Law 9.433/97 is an indirectly constitutional rule of restriction. For, to repeat Robert Alexy, every time ordinary laws are referred to as restrictions, a competence is established to impose said restrictions.

Having established the premise that Law 9.433/97 acts as a restrictive rule for a fundamental right, it is not difficult to see that charging for water is also a restriction on a fundamental right. Charging limits the free use of water by people and entities. If charging is also a way of restricting a fundamental right, then it can only be done by law, as Robert Alexy observed when he defined restrictions on fundamental rights as norms.

Thus, given that it is a fundamental right, as has been said, but also that the asset is a limited and exhaustible environmental resource, the attribution of economic value was inevitable. This will seek to impress upon the user the notion of the "real value" of water, which should not be limited to the quantification of a monetary value, seen from the perspective of utilitarianism, but, above all, a value linked to the very existence of life in the world.

Paulo Afonso Leme Machado rightly states that:

> Water is now measured in terms of economic values. This cannot and should not lead to conduct that allows anyone to use water at will by paying a fee. Valuing water must take into account the importance of conserving, restoring and better distributing this good[216].

As you can see, the economic valuation of water makes it possible to recognize, beyond

---

[216] MACHADO, Paulo Afonso Leme. Resources ..., p. 32.

the monetary value, the need to preserve and recover water for present and future generations. In this sense, the National Water Resources Policy carefully determines that the funds collected from charging for water resources will not only be used to finance studies, programs, projects and works related specifically to water resources, but will above all be used in the hydrographic basin in which they were generated. In other words, the cost of water finances its preservation and recovery. Let's look at the wording of art. 22 of Law 9.433/97:

> Art. 22: The amounts collected from charging for the use of water resources shall be applied as a priority in the hydrographic basin in which they were generated and will be used:
> I - in the financing of studies, programs, projects and works included in the Water Resources Plans;
> II - to pay for the implementation and administrative costs of the bodies and entities that make up the National Water Resources Management System.
> § Paragraph 1. The application to the expenses provided for in item II of this article is limited to seven and a half percent of the total collected.
> § Paragraph 2 - The amounts provided for in the *main* body of this article may be applied on a non-repayable basis to projects and works that alter the quality, quantity and flow regime of a body of water in a way considered beneficial to the community.

As you can see, the implementation of public policies for the rational use, preservation and recovery of water resources can only achieve the desired results if the financial resources for this are sufficient to engage in pro-active behavior. It is not difficult to see that public bodies, faced with a shortage of resources, first undertake corrective activities, in the sense that once the damage has been verified, they try to correct it. Preventive activities (such as environmental education) are left to one side until sufficient resources have been allocated.

In the French model, the contribution of financial resources is significant, so much so that the policies for restoring water sources are intensive[217] . This attitude is a strong example

---

[217] It's enough to note that in France, charging allows the recovery of water sources. "Charging by French water agencies since 1969 has led to an increase in the number of urban water treatment plants, from around 64 at the start of the 1960s to around 260 in 1970. Today, around 1,900 urban water treatment plants are in operation throughout France. Through the resources collected from the clean-up charge, the water agencies have financed, free of charge, the investments needed to comply with the five-year programs approved by the Basin Committees." Author not identified. Hydrographic basins: new management of water resources. Available at: http://www.eco.umcamp.br/ecoeco/artigos/encontros/downloads/mesa3/3.pdf#search='batias%20hidrogr%C3%

to follow.

6.3. The polluter pays principle.

Since charging is a restriction on a fundamental right, which implies that it must be enshrined in law, we are moving in the direction of charging for water being instrumentalized through taxation. In environmental law, the rule that strongly supports environmental taxation is the polluter pays principle, and it is necessary to make a brief incursion into its origin and function in the environmental order.

The "polluter-pays principle"[218] was introduced by the Organization for Economic Cooperation and Development in 1972, with the adoption of Recommendation C(72)128 of the Directing Council, which dealt with the economic aspects of environmental policies, recognizing that the market could not act freely to the detriment of environmental quality[219].

The polluter pays principle recognizes that environmental resources are scarce and that their use in production and consumption leads to their reduction and degradation[220]. If the market does not recognize the cost of reducing environmental resources in its prices, the problem of scarcity will not be internalized by the production system. "From an economic point of view, it is as if a price were created for the use of environmental resources, because, on the contrary, if a zero cost is adopted for this exploitation, waste is certain in the face of a false impression of abundance or infinity"[221].

Therefore, this principle is best understood through its purpose, which is to achieve

---

Alficas%20nova%20gest%C3%A3o%20de%20reursos%20h%C3%ADdricos. Accessed on: July 2, 2005.

[218] SEBASTIAO, Simone Martins. Tributo ..., p. 210.

[219] ANTUNES, Paulo de Bessa. Direito ..., p. 42. GUERRA, Sidney. International Environmental Law. Rio de Janeiro: Maria Augusta Delgado, 2006, p. 79.

[220] ANTUNES, Paulo de Bessa. op. cit., p. 42.

[221] SEBASTIAO, Simone Martins. Tributo..., p. 214.

greater care in relation to the polluting potential of production, in the search for a satisfactory quality of the environment.

Cleucio Santos Nunes warns that

> economic production, in some sectors, brings with it the destruction of the environment. This is a well-known fact; if it weren't, there would be no reason for the development of environmental law. It is neither fair nor just that the cost of this destruction should be shared by society as a whole, with the polluter having no specific onus in the distribution of environmental losses[222] .

The aim is for the social costs that accompany the production process to be internalized, i.e. for economic agents to take them into account when drawing up their production costs and therefore assume them.

Cristiane Derani teaches that

> During the production process, in addition to the product to be sold, 'negative externalities' are produced. These are called externalities because, although they result from production, they are received by the community, unlike profit, which is perceived by the private producer. Hence the expression 'privatization of profits and socialization of losses', when negative externalities are identified. With the application of the polluter pays principle, an attempt is made to correct this added cost to society by imposing its internalization. This is why this principle is also known as the principle of responsibility[223] .

Given these considerations, it is clear that this constitutional principle[224] (art. 225, §3, in its modern interpretation that must escape the cause-effect logic) imposes on those who cause contamination to suffer economically unfavorable consequences, either through taxes (as a source of funds for environmental protection), whose taxable event must be related to the fact of contamination; or through other legal instruments[225] , such as the imposition of fines, environmental licensing, determination of environmental clean-up and recovery[226] .

---

[222] NUNES, Cleucio Santos. Law ..., p. 49-50.

[223] DERANI, Cristiane. Economic Environmental Law. Sao Paulo: Max Limonad, 1997, p. 158.

[224] The treaty establishing a constitution for Europe, currently under discussion, states in its Section 5 - Environment, Article III-233, number 2: "The Union's policy on the environment shall aim to achieve a high level of protection, taking into account the diversity of situations in the various regions of the Union. It is based on the principles of precaution and preventive action, on the principle that environmental damage should, as a priority, be rectified at source and on the principle that the polluter pays".

[225] TABOADA, Carlos Palao El principio "quien contamina paga" y el principio de capacidad economica. In: Direito Tributario Ambiental. org. Heleno Taveira Torres. Sao Paulo: Malheiros, 2005, p.94.

[226] OLIVEIRA, Jose Marcos Domingues. Direito Tributario e Meio Ambiente: proporcionalidade, tipicidade aberta, afetagao da receita. Rio de Janeiro: Renovar, 1999, p. 25.

Cleucio Santos Nunes observes that "it is through this principle that measures such as the imposition of environmental taxes ('ecotaxes') have been used in various countries around the world, and even - albeit very tentatively - in Brazil."[227] .

For, as Antonio Herman V. Benjamin rightly pointed out, when he highlighted the reasons for adopting instruments such as taxes, with a view to sharing social burdens,

> by the end of the 1960s, it was clear that traditional legal remedies, of a privatistic nature, were not capable of halting or reducing the growing degradation of the planet's natural resources: a typical case of "market failure", in which case state intervention would be required to combat environmental extremities[228] .

But these impositions of protectionist measures are not without other social costs, as they can serve to increase social exclusion to the extent that the cost of the final product can leave certain social groups on the margins of consumption. Cleucio Santos Nunes explains:

> The imposition of economic burdens (taxation is one example), as instruments to make the principle effective, results in an increase in the cost of the good produced, which can generate distortions in the market. The main - and cruelest - of these is the exclusion of layers of less well-off consumers who can't afford to pay the cost added to the product by the environmental tax burden - which generates more social and economic inequality, especially in countries with unequal income distribution, as is the case in Brazil. Another consequence - and this one seems very remote, because the market has its automatic adjustment mechanisms - would be a freezing of the means of exchange, to the extent that prices could reach unpayable levels.
>
> Given these variables, two developments of the polluter pays principle emerge as alternatives to be adopted, depending on the local characteristics of each market. These are "the sharing of social burdens and environmental losses by the exploitative economic process and the use of the polluter pays principle as an instrument to guide public environmental policies that reduce ecological damage".[229]

Thus, as can be seen, *it is precisely* in the provision of the polluter-pays principle that the legislator finds grounds to use environmental taxes effectively in environmental protection, as they exert a strong coercive power over the citizen. "Taxes have a social character and their

---

227 NUNES, Cleucio Santos. Tax law and the environment. Sao Paulo: Dialetica, 2005, p. 50.
228 BENJAMIN, Antonio Herman V. O Estado Teatral e a implementação do direito ambiental. *In:* 7th International Congress of Environmental Law - "Law, Water and Life", 7, 2003, Sao Paulo. p. 348.
229 NUNES, Cleucio Santos. Tax law and the environment. Sao Paulo: Dialetica, 2005, p. 50.

flexibility allows them to be used more intensively to protect the environment."[230] .

In Brazil, the experience of environmental taxation is in its infancy, despite the fact that the Federal Constitution has provided the legislator with a wide range of possibilities for exercising extrafiscal powers, with the polluter pays principle being an irrefutable foundation for instituting environmental taxation.

6.4. Extrafiscal function of the tax.

When dealing with the function of taxes, especially in the environmental field, we enter into a debate that must necessarily address taxation and extrafiscality, as well as the destination of tax revenue. The Federal Constitution brings back to tax law the analysis of the role of the destination of revenue when it introduces the figure of special contributions and removes the incidence in this area of art. 4 of the National Tax Code.

It is true that the primary purpose of instituting taxes is to raise funds to achieve the objectives chosen by the government, as well as to fulfill its institutional purpose, although there are those who maintain that taxation is a rule of social rejection and is often at the service not of the public interest or of society, but functions as an instrument for keeping those in power in power[231] .

But the fiscal function is not the only function of taxation. Especially in the field of Environmental Law, extrafiscality has been debated, as this function directs the tax towards purposes other than raising money for the Treasury[232] , inducing behavior in order to stimulate

---

[230] RIBAS, Lidia Maria Lopes Rodrigues. Environmental defense: use of tax instruments. ". In Direito Tributario Ambiental. org. Heleno Taveira Torres. Sao Paulo: Malheiros, 2005, p. 685.
[231] MARTINS, Ives Gandra da Silva. A theory of Taxation. Sao Paulo: Quartier Latin, 2005, p. 51.
[232] OLIVEIRA, .ГсБё Marcos Domingues. Law ..., p. 38.

or discourage conduct in line with the social, political and economic objectives of the State[233] .

Thus, in the field of environmental law, taxation emerges as an instrument capable of preventing and combating pollution, both by means of a reward sanction, taxing less severely those who don't pollute or pollute relatively little (in this sense the extra-fiscal function comes to the fore)[234] , such as by imposing a tax "ex lege" so that the polluter internalizes or bears the cost of the general or specific public services necessary for environmental preservation and recovery or for environmental inspection and monitoring[235] . Hence the diagnosis by Marcos Domingues de Oliveira:

> The tax system can act as a complement to the administrative system of environmental licenses, which is indispensable for preventing and combating pollution; it is also useful for preserving environmental resources, by adapting tax species to environmental taxation.[236]

An important aspect of extrafiscality is that, by choosing to give the tax a function other than collection, the legislator no longer uses contributory capacity[237] as the basis for distinctions and, according to some scholars, starts using proportionality. This is why Tc3ë Marcos Domingues de Oliveira argues that police fees, for example, can exceed the exact cost of the inspection activity, as a way of discouraging conduct harmful to the environment[238] .

However, the issue is not without controversy, as some scholars argue that extrafiscality is only a matter for taxes.

Marco Aurelio Greco believes that extrafiscality can take on a positive meaning of providing a stimulus, facilitating the development of an activity, and a negative meaning of discouraging or hindering a certain activity. The author recognizes that the Constitution itself sometimes allows extrafiscal functions in both directions, as can be seen in relation to IPI and

---

[233] SEBASTIAO, Simone Martins. Environmental Taxation. Curitiba: Jurua, 2006, p. 133.
[234] OLIVEIRA, Josë Marcos Domingues. op. cit., p. 39.
[235] Ibid., p. 42.
[236] Ibid., p. 44.
[237] SEBASTIAO, Simone Martins. Tributo ..., p. 136.
[238] OLIVEIRA, .Teбë Marcos Domingues. Law..., p. 60-61.

ICMS. However, it rules out its occurrence in relation to special contributions. In his words:

> extrafiscality is not a concept that, in my opinion, is relevant when examining contributions, including intervention contributions. In these cases, the profile of the requirement is different and collection is not a parameter for gauging the meaning and function of the requirement. Contributions don't exist on the basis of collection, but on the basis of the purpose for which they are intended. Even if it were intended to apply the concept of extrafiscality to contributions, it would be forgiving to recognize, for the reasons explained above, that in relation to them, extrafiscality could only assume a positive and not a negative function.

This conception is in line with the National Water Resources Policy, which, alongside the grant, institutes water charges - which, as will be shown, is a contribution to intervene in the economic domain - as a coercive instrument, simultaneously raising funds for the recovery and preservation of water bodies; inducing conduct that preserves the quantity and quality of water resources; and users internalizing the social costs added to the economic activity they carry out.

6.5. *Immunity from existential minimum.*

The theory of the existential minimum in connection with first-generation fundamental rights developed in post-war Germany in the face of the deficiency of the Bonn Charter,[239] which did not include fundamental rights of a social nature. "The German Constitutional Court drew the right to a 'minimum standard of existence' from the principle of human dignity (Article 1, I, Basic Law) and from the right to life and physical integrity, through a systematic

---

[239] KRELL, Andreas J. Direitos sociais e controle judicial no Brasil e na Alemanha: os (des)caminhos de um direito constitucional "comparado". Porto Alegre: Sergio Antonio Fabris Editor, 2002, p. 60.

interpretation in conjunction with the principle of the welfare state."[240] .

There is a right to minimum conditions of dignified human existence that cannot be the object of state intervention. This right is directly related to the rights to freedom, equality, due process of law and free enterprise, as well as involving the idea of justice and the redistribution of social wealth, according to Ricardo Lobo Torres[241] . The basis of the right to a minimum standard of living would be "the conditions for the exercise of freedom, which some authors include in real freedom, positive freedom or even pure freedom, in order to differentiate it from freedom that is merely the absence of constraint"[242] .

The right to a minimum is not expressly stated in the Brazilian Federal Constitution, although it derives from the principles it adopts, such as the principle of proportionality. It is also not enshrined in Western Constitutions, with the exception of Canada's. It is more often found in international declarations, such as the Universal Declaration of Human Rights of 1948 and the Declaration on the Right to Development (UN, 1986).

The right to existential minimum has no defined content, it appears as general clauses and indeterminate types, and is not exhausted by the list in Article 5 of the Constitution[243] . Political, economic and social rights can also find protection in the protection of the existential minimum insofar as, if they are not met, they lead to the denial of a dignified existence for human beings[244] . Therefore, according to Luis Roberto Barroso, "even if the values could oscillate significantly according to what each person considers to be the minimum standard of dignity, the fact is that there is a central core on which there will be consensus in any

---

[240] Ibid., p. 61.
[241] TORRES, Ricardo Lobo. The existential minimum and fundamental rights. *In:* Revista de Direito Administrativo, n. 177: 29-49, Sao Paulo: FGVEditora, jul./set., 1989, p. 29.
[242] Ibid., p. 30.
[243] TORRES, Ricardo Lobo. The minimum..., p. 32-33.
[244] "If we add to this that precisely the idea of fundamental rights is that the things which are especially important to the individual and which can be legally guaranteed should be so..." (ALEXY, Robert. Teoria de los Derechos ..., p. 488-489).

circumstance"[245] .

It would be agreed, then, that the "minimum social standard" would "always include basic and efficient health care, access to basic food and clothing, primary education and guaranteed housing; the concrete content of this minimum, however, will vary from country to country"[246] .

Fernando Facury Scaff warns that

> It's imperative to note that the concept of existential minimum, anchored in the primacy of freedom, should have greater scope in those countries on the periphery of capitalism. After all, only those who have the capacity to exercise freedom can fully exercise it, even within the scope of the existential minimum. And for this exercise of legal freedom to be possible, it is necessary to ensure real freedom (Alexy), or the possibility of exercising one's capacities (Amartya), through fundamental social rights[247] .

The Supreme Court of the United States, however, considers that the right to a minimum standard of living does not affect economic and social rights, such as the right to education or housing, "making a strong argument that 'poverty and immorality' are not synonymous"[248] , thus not allowing social rights to be subject to judicial review.

Indeed, for Ricardo Lobo Torres, the problem of the existential minimum would be addressed to the prohibition of the state allowing the absolute poverty of the individual, which cannot be defined due to the fluidity of its concept[249] , and it is certain that, if the possibility of survival is affected, the right to the existential minimum is under attack.

In tax law, the *status negativus of* the existential minimum is affirmed through tax immunities, to the extent that tax imposition, like the ability to pay, does not allow invasion of

---

[245] BARROSO, Luis Roberto. O Direito constitucional e a efetividade de suas normas - limites e possiblidade da Constituigao brasileira. 7. ed., Rio de Janeiro: Renovar, 2003, p. 153.
[246] KRELL, Andreas J. Direitos ..., p. 63.
[247] SCAFF, Fernando Facury. Reserve of the possible, existential minimum and human rights. *In:* Principles of

Pires and Heleno Taveira Torres (organizers), Rio de Janeiro: Renovar, 2006, p. 122.
TORRES, Ricardo Lobo. O minimo ..., p. 34.
Ibid., p. 30.

[248]

the sphere of the citizen's minimum freedom represented by the right to subsistence. Without major problems in water law, the manifestation of the existential minimum, given the importance of this element for the subsistence of life, is incontrovertible, especially when debating the right of access to water for human consumption and animal watering (defined as a priority in situations of scarcity by Law 9.433/97, art. 1, inc. III).

The effects of the theory of the existential minimum on taxation are evident insofar as the right to the existential minimum[250] prohibits the imposition of taxes on the core essential to maintaining a dignified life. This is true tax immunity because it derives directly from the core of fundamental rights and, together with the ability to pay, prevents unfair and non-solidary taxation.

> The immunity of the existential minimum falls short of the ability to pay, in the same way that the prohibition of confiscation prevents taxation beyond the ability to pay. In other words, the ability to pay comes before the minimum necessary for a dignified human existence and ends before the destructive limit of property[251] .

Ricardo Lobo Torres warns that it doesn't matter if the immunity of the existential minimum appears in the legislation in the form of an exemption[252] , because what truly characterizes immunity is not the label by which it is taxed in some piece of legislation, but the fact that it finds its true substrate in the nuclei of fundamental rights from which the rule prohibiting attacks on the minimum for the existence of human beings is drawn. On this point, the understanding espoused here departs from that of Ricardo Lobo Torres, who believes that the foundation of the existential minimum is pre-constitutional and is a predicate of the right to freedom. On the contrary, we believe that it is not only pre-constitutional, but also a

---

[250] "Income tax is not levied on a minimum essential to the survival of the declarant, nor on the amounts necessary for the subsistence of his dependents, deductible at source. This is immunity from the existential minimum..." (TORRES, Ricardo Lobo. O minimo ..., p. 36.).

[251] TORRES, Ricardo Lobo. Treatise on constitutional financial and tax law - human rights and taxation: immunities and isonomy. 3. ed. Revised and updated up to December 31, 2003, the date of publication of Constitutional Amendment no. 42 of December 19, 2003. Rio de Janeiro: Renovar, 2005, p. 187.

[252] TORRES, Ricardo Lobo. O minimo ..., p. 36.

constitutional norm, insofar as immunity also derives from the principles adopted by the Constitution (art. 5, § 2 of the Charter of the Republic).

The existential minimum would then be a right protected negatively against state intervention and, at the same time, guaranteed positively by state services. In Brazil, the immunity of the existential minimum has been misinterpreted, being based on the ability to pay. However, it is in the non-contributory capacity that the initributability of the right to existential minimum is manifested. In fact, the ability to pay presupposes economic potential[253] , but it does not necessarily mean that the taxpayer will have the economic availability to pay the tax. Contributory capacity is given by that part of a person's economic potential, of their wealth, which exceeds the minimum subsistence level, which is why the implicit constitutional immunity of the minimum subsistence level comes before the manifestation of economic capacity[254] . In the words of Ricardo Lobo Torres:

> The initial conditions of freedom and the non-taxability of the minimum subsistence level, therefore, coincide with non-contributory capacity, which is the negative side of the principle that appears positively in the Constitution. The existential minimum finds its basis in the ability to pay and never its foundation. Both are part of the same equation of values, in contrast to the interaction between freedom and justice, ideas in which they are intertwined[255] .

Therefore, in the case of water, where it is immediately clear that it is essential to the existence of life, its protection is part of the protection of the existential minimum, which is why a tax that seeks to take away the individual's ability to consume water for their subsistence is unacceptable.

---

[253] GRUPENMACHER, Betina Treiger. Fiscal justice and existential minimum. *In:* Principios de direito financeiro e tributario - estudos em homenagem ao Professor Ricardo Lobo Torres. Adilson Rodrigues Pires and Heleno Taveira Torres (organizers), Rio de Janeiro: Renovar, 2006, p.108.

[254] "Systems that take into account the principle of ability to pay impose taxation only on the disposable income of natural and legal persons for the payment of taxes, this principle implying an absolute prohibition of taxation on income necessary for survival." (Ibid., p.109).

[255] TORRES, Ricardo Lobo. Tratado de direito constitucional financeiro e tributario - os direitos humanos e a tributação: imunidades e isonomia..., p. 187.

With regard to the existential minimum, it is also necessary to verify whether water is situated as a right to the minimum necessary for survival or under the protection of the ecological minimum. This is because the protection of the subsistence minimum prevents taxation as long as there is no ability to pay and the protection of the ecological minimum means that the government is obliged to invest budgetary funds in the environment in order to implement sustainable development.

Internationalists have also mentioned the right to sustainable development as a human right[256] . There are aspects of the right to development that are essentially linked to fundamental rights, such as the minimum necessary for existence (basic education, preventive health, drinking water, etc.) and the ecological minimum (a healthy environment) .[257]

"Sustainable human development" has an intimate relationship with a healthy environment and the rights of future generations, which is why it places people at the center of development and emphasizes that today's inequalities are so great that to sustain the present form of development is to perpetuate similar inequalities for future generations. The right to human development or the principle of sustainable human development, therefore, becomes extraordinarily important for the issue of the minimum existential, because it postulates the obligatory budgetary expenditure for the guarantee of the status *positivus libertatis.*

It should be noted that, for Ricardo Lobo Torres, the right to drinking water is part of the right to the vital minimum and not the ecological minimum. This is because this environmental resource is essential for life. However, to the extent that the need to consume water goes beyond vital needs, water resources gain the protection of the ecological minimum, as an essential good for the maintenance and preservation of ecosystems.

---

[256] "International agreements on human rights are marked by the need to promote development as a solution to poverty and as a guarantor of equality. The environment itself is considered a human right in these treaties, especially in the more anthropocentric cultures. In this way, the concepts of human rights (purpose) are united with the concepts of environmental law (conditionality) and economic development (economic growth), giving rise to the concept of economic development". (VARELLA, Marcelo Dias. Direito international..., p. 40).

[257] TORRES, Ricardo Lobo. Tratado de direito constitucional financeiro e tributario - os direitos humanos e a tributação: imunidades e isonomia. ..., p. 173.

From this perspective of protecting the ecological minimum, the reverse emerges - not initributability, not non-contributory capacity - but the manifestation of economic potentiality, a presupposition of contributory capacity. This is not to identify the 'ability to affect' the environment with the ability to pay, which would be a distortion of this principle[258] , because the use of environmental goods is not, in itself, an index of economic capacity, but the connection between the use of the environment and the objective manifestation of economic capacity is irrefutable.

In fact, it is in economic activity - which exploits environmental resources for uses other than those intended to provide the bare minimum of life for each individual - that the greatest "contaminating capacity"[259] manifests itself, and it is in this "contaminating capacity" that the economic substrate of economic activity resides. Unreasonable consumer activity, beyond that aimed at providing the minimum subsistence level, also damages the environment.

It should be noted that it is the performance of economic activity that has the greatest impact on the environment. In this sense, the ecological minimum becomes yet another foundation for taxation in its extra-fiscal form, so as to allow taxation to have the function of protecting and preserving the environment, striving to achieve compatibility between development and the land ethic[260] , or rather, the right to sustainable development.

---

[258] "the economic force legitimizing the subject's aptitude to contribute would not come from the subject's 'capacity' or 'aptitude' to influence the environment, in itself considered, i.e. from the utilization of the environment, but of the economic substrate, manifestation of economic force, from which the environment is affected', i.e. the economic activities causing the contamination - which must be distinguished, we note, from the contaminating action itself; es decir, emision o vertido -, o incluso los bienes o instalaciones mediante los cuales se realiza dicha actividad". (TABOADA, Carlos Palao. El principio "quien contamina paga" y el principio de capacidad economica. In Direto Tributario Ambiental. org. Heleno Taveira Torres. Sao Paulo: Malheiros, 2005, p.91).

[259] "That is to say, the object of the tax would be the 'contaminating capacity', not as such a capacity in itself considered, but as an expression of the existence of an income, patrimony or consumption from which it would be contaminated; these elements of economic reality assuming the function of object of the tax". (TABOADA, Carlos Palao. El principio..., p 93).

[260] "Land ethics is based on an attitude of respect for nature because of its intrinsic value and not because of the instrumental value it has for human beings." (CARVALHO, Edson Ferreira de. Meio ..., p. 323).

6.6. *Taxation and water.*

As the various items in this chapter have shown, a powerful instrument at the service of environmental preservation is taxation. Its coercive force is significantly effective in preventing the degradation of the environment and especially water.

The economic theories of Arthur Pigou and Vilfredo Pareto; the need to find a new holistic ethics, capable of leading the Law to broaden its atomistic conception, centered solely on the human person; the theory of fundamental rights, which states that any restriction on a fundamental right must be imposed by law; the extrafiscal function of taxation; the theory of the existential minimum and the ecological minimum provide the necessary theoretical support for the interpretation of articles 19 and following of Law 9.433/97. 19 et seq. of Law 9.433/97, in the sense of taxing water charges.

These grounds, together with the fact that, as will be shown below, the elements of the water charge constitute the main rule of a contribution to intervene in the economic domain, impose the tax nature of the charge.

Indeed, if taxation is the best way to preserve water and if restrictions on the fundamental right of access to water can only be established by law, which must respect, as in fact it did, the vital minimum, then the levy could not have any other legal nature, otherwise it would be blatantly unconstitutional.

Chapter 7

Water charges: tax or public service?

7.1. Overcoming the classic view.

The new legal discipline for water raises a number of doubts about the institute of charging. Now, without further reflection, when we are dealing with the use of an essential natural resource, which does not necessarily involve the provision of a public service, we immediately refer to the figure of the public price to qualify such a charge. Consuelo Yoshida considers that

> Strictly speaking, it can be seen from the legislation that regulates the matter that this is a compulsory charge for the use of an essential natural resource, which does not necessarily involve the provision of a public service, the definition of values of which is not freely governed by market laws. It is because of these hybrid characteristics that it is difficult to characterize the requirement as a price (because it is a legal imposition in the cases where it is required) or as a fee (because it is a consideration, remuneration, compensation for the use of a natural resource, without the provision

of a public service)[261] .

On the other hand, this conclusion that the use of a natural resource results in a public charge is difficult to overcome when we see that the charge is not governed freely by the laws of the market and is not based on a contract, but is an "ex lege" obligation imposed on all users who, in carrying out some economic activity, may generate pollution, harmful alterations to the level of the water body, etc.

In addition, the fact that the law has linked the funds collected to a legal purpose of guaranteeing the preservation of water resources (art. 2 combined with articles 6 and 7 combined with arts. 19 and 22 all of Law 9.433/97), as well as the fact that the financial resources are linked to the hydrographic basin in which they are generated (with Law 9.984/2000 providing for a different way of accounting for these resources, in a way excepting the principle of the unity of the treasury), reveal that classifying the collection as a public service is no longer such an obvious task[262] .

In fact, if we look at the examples of France, Germany and Spain, we can see that, in these countries, the charge instituted has been qualified by doctrine as a tax.

It must also be argued that, from a brief analysis of the Water Code, Law 9.433/97 represents a paradigm shift. In fact, the 1934 legislation does not tie the charging of water to any specific purpose, nor does it tie the collection of the amounts to the fulfillment of any purpose, but only considers that, according to the convenience and opportunity of the

---

[261] YOSHIDA, Consuelo Yatsuda Moromizato. The effectiveness and environmental efficiency of economic, economic-financial and tax instruments. Emphasis on prevention. The economic use of environmental goods and its implications. In Direito Tributario Ambiental. org. Heleno Taveira Torres. Sao Paulo: Malheiros, 2005, p.558-559.

[262] In the opposite direction, understanding that charging is a public charge: DANTAS, Fabiana Santos. Water Resources Management: a critical analysis of Law 9.433/97. *In:* The application of environmental law in the federal state. Adreas J. Krell (org.) Rio de Janeiro: Editora Lumens Juris, 2005, p. 309. POMPEU, Cid Tomanik. Water law in Brazil. São Paulo: Editora Revista dos Tribunais, 2006, p. 279. GRANZIERA, Maria Luiza Machado. Water law: legal discipline of fresh waters. São Paulo: Atlas, 2001, p. 224. MACHADO, Paulo Affonso Leme. Water resources - Brazilian and international law. São Paulo: Malheiros Ediotres, 2002, p. 88. VIEGAS, Eduardo Coral. Legal Vision of Water. Porto Alegre: Livraria do Advogado, 2005, p.109. FARIAS, Paulo Josë Leite. Water: economic or ecological legal asset? Brasilia: Brasilia Juridica, 2005, p. 440.

administrative district to which the water belongs (Union, State or Municipality), the use may be free or remunerated (art. 36 of the Water Code).

The environmental doctrine seems to agree that charging is a public charge[263] . There is no mention of an *ex lege* obligation, *there is* no consideration of the purpose pursued by the institute, nor is there any link between the amounts collected and the purposes legally pursued.

The problem with not attributing a tax nature to the collection, in the environmental doctrine, lies in the fact that it is still attached to the concepts of the science of Financial Law, which classifies income into the public coffers as originating and derived revenue, a classification that is irrelevant to the science of Tax Law. In fact, in order to attribute a tax nature to a given legal fact, the starting point is something else, not Financial Law. This problem, now largely overcome by tax doctrine, used to occur when classifying the "generating event"[264] into tax species, or rather, classifying the hypothesis of incidence, as Paulo de Barros Carvalho warned:

> The passage of time and the gradual detachment of the science of tax law from the economic categories that illuminated it have gradually demonstrated the deficiency of the underlying belief in that classification[265] .

All the authors who propose to attribute the legal nature of a public charge to water charges begin by informing the reader of their works that there are two types of revenue, originating and derived, and then, considering that it is an originating revenue, conclude that the charge is not a tax, just to mention those works that deal specifically with water. In environmental law courses, the scientific panorama is even worse, since, as a rule, the subject is not even mentioned or, if it is mentioned, it is not developed. Strictly speaking, the concept

---

[263] Paulo Bessa Antunes, Maria Luiza Machado Granziera, Paulo Afonso Leme, Paulo -ГсБё Leite Farias, Celso Antonio Fiorilo, Cid Tomanik Pompeu.

[264] Nomenclature that has only brought atechnicality to the science of Tax Law, as pondered by Geraldo Ataliba, who introduces the notion of hypothesis of incidence.

[265] CARVALHO, Paulo de Barros. Teoria da Norma Tributaria. Sao Paulo: Max Limonad, 1998, p. 178.

of tax is not broken down in order to check whether its constituent elements are present in the charge. That's what we'll do next.

When Law 9.433/97 is approached in the light of tax doctrine, the issue takes on new contours. Analyzing charging under the theory of tax law reveals some peculiarities that cannot be ignored when establishing the legal regime of this category.

Ricardo Lobo Torres states that the charging of water, in the form of participation in the results of exploitation (art. 20, §1 combined with art. 176, §2 of CF/88), financial compensation (art. 20, §1 of CF/88 combined with art. 17 Law 9.648/98 and art. 28 of Law 9.984/00) and various tariffs for the use of water resources (art. 17, inc. II and §2 of Law 9.648/98), takes on the character of a public charge. Although this study does not analyze the nature of art. 19 et seq. of Law 9.433/97, it does recognize that "industrial or collective consumption and the abstraction and use of sources and springs are also done free of charge, although they give rise to a public charge, which will be levied on the cost/benefit of providing the public service and not on the public good"[266] , thus demonstrating that it is not the use that justifies the charge.

On the other hand, Heleno Taveira Torres recognizes in art. 19 of Law 9.433/97 a true contribution of intervention in the economic domain:

> It is found in Law 9.433, of 8.1.1997, which establishes the policy of water resources, when the "granting of rights to use water resources" was created, provided for in art. 19 of that law, which we understand as a typical type of CIDE, despite the irregularities presented, such as the lack of definition of the rates, which was left to ANA Resolutions, in direct affront to the principle of legality[267] .

The case law of the higher courts has yet **to** analyze conflicts in the light of the new legislation (Law 9.433/97). However, there are a large number of precedents from the Superior

---

[266] TORRES, Ricardo Lobo. The taxation of public services in the State of the risk society. In Public Services and Tax Law. TORRES, Heleno Taveira (coordination). Sao Paulo: Quartier Latin, 2005, p. 136.
[267] TORRES, Heleno Taveira. The relationship ..., p. 108.

Court of Justice which hold that charging for water and sewage is a service fee[268].

On the other hand, it must be recognized that the National Water Agency has been charging for water on the basis of a single basic price, set by the National Water Resources Council. This does not in itself mean that the charge created by Article 19 et seq. of Law 9.433/97 is a public charge and not a tax. It is up to the legal operator to analyze the figure created by law and establish a legal regime for it.

This phenomenon of disguising real taxes with the mask of public charges is not unique to the Brazilian state, with Herrera Molina and Carbajo Vasco diagnosing that in Spain "various figures of a predominantly taxing nature are emerging - even though the legislator calls them 'canons' - whose structure nevertheless has some of the characteristics of taxes (this

---

[268] TAX. WATER SUPPLY AND SEWAGE COLLECTION SERVICES. TAX. TAXABLE NATURE. PRECEDENTS. (1) The service of water supply and sewage collection is charged to the user by the supplying entity as a fee, when it is compulsory. (2) In this case, it is a public service granted, of a compulsory nature, in order to meet collective or public needs. 3. There is no legal support for the thesis that the difference between a fee and a public charge derives from the nature of the relationship established between the consumer or user and the entity providing or supplying the good or service, so that if the entity providing the service is governed by public law, the amount charged would be characterized as a fee, since the relationship between the two is governed by public law; on the other hand, if the provider of the public service is a legal person governed by private law, the amount charged is a public charge/fee. 4) Prevalence in the legal system of the conclusions of the X National Symposium on Tax Law, to the effect that "the legal nature of the remuneration derives from the essence of the activity carried out, and is not affected by the existence of the concession. The concession holder receives remuneration of the same nature as that which the Granting Authority would receive if it provided the service directly". (RF, July to September 1987, year 1987, v. 299, page 40). 5. (5) Article 11 of Law No. 2.312/94 (National Health Code) states: "It is compulsory for every building considered habitable to be connected to a sewage system, the effluent of which will have a destination set by the competent authority". 6 Compulsory water and sewage service. Essential public activity (service) made available to the community for its well-being and health protection. 7) "Water and sewage services are normally paid for by means of a fee, given the compulsory connection of households to the public network" (Helly Lopes Meirelles, in "Direito Municipal Brasileiro", 3ª ed., RT - 1977, page 492). 8) "If the legal order obliges the use of a certain service, not allowing the respective need to be met by another means, then it is fair that the corresponding remuneration, charged by the Government, should suffer the limitations proper to a tax". (Hugo de Brito Machado, in "Regime Tributario da Venda de Agua", Rev. Jurid. da Procuradoria-Geral da Fazenda Estadual/Minas Gerais, no. 05, page 11). 9. 9) Adoption of the thesis, in the specific situation examined, that the contribution for the supply of water and sewage collection is a fee. 10 - Precedents of the 1stª and 2ndª Panels of this Superior Court. (REsp 818649, DJ 02.05.2006 p. 273) . STJ Precedents: - RESP 167489-SP (RSTJ 112/89, RDR 14/201), RESP 453855-MS, RESP 495387-PR (RSTJ 176/268), RESP 480692-MS (RET 33/39), RESP 439570-DF (RJADCOAS 45/96, RSTJ 173/125). TAX. SEWAGE SERVICE. LEGAL NATURE OF REMUNERATION. TAX. COMPULSORY USE. SUBJECT TO THE TAX REGIME. DOMINANT STJ ORIENTATION. SPECIAL APPEAL DISMISSED. 1 The dominant case law of this Court considers that the amount demanded as consideration for the water and sewage service has the legal nature of a fee - and is therefore subject to the legal regime of taxation, especially with regard to compliance with the principle of legality - whenever it is used compulsorily, regardless of whether it is carried out directly by the Government or by a concessionaire. 2. special appeal dismissed (REsp 782270, DJ 07.11.2005 p. 163).

is the case of the autonomous sanitation canons)"[269] .

In national doctrine, Hugo de Brito Machado detects these circumstances where, instead of instituting a tax, it is disguised as if it were a pecuniary payment demanded without respect for the rules and principles that make up the legal system of taxation, which he calls a hidden tax[270] .

7.2. *Identification of the rights to use water resources that can be charged for.*

In order to define the legal regime to which charging is subordinate, it is necessary to know which rights to use water resources are grantable, since the legal text (art. 20 of Law 9.433/97[271]) links and subordinates charging to granting, as interdependent instruments. Therefore, according to the legal system, only the use that can be granted will be charged.

The purpose of licensing is to control the quantity and quality of water in order to harmonize its multiple uses.

At this point, the Water Law lists some uses that will be subject to licensing, including (sections I to IV of art. 12) 12): the derivation or abstraction of a portion of the water in a body of water for final consumption, including public supply, or as an input in a production process; the extraction of water from a subterranean aquifer for final consumption or as an input in a production process; the discharge into a body of water of sewage and other liquid or gaseous waste, whether treated or not, for the purposes of dilution, transportation or final disposal; the

---

[269] MOLINA, Pedro Manuel Herrera; and VASCO, Carbajo Domingo. Marco conceptual, constituional y comunitario de la fiscalidad ecologica. In: Direito Tributario Ambiental. org. Heleno Taveira Torres. Sao Paulo: Malheiros, 2005, p. 168.

[270] MACHADO, Hugo de Brito. Public Services and Taxation. *In:* Public Services and Tax Law. Heleno Taveira Torres (coord.) Sao Paulo: Quartier Latin, 2005, p. 282.

[271] Art. 20: Charges will be levied for the use of water resources subject to granting, under the terms of article 12 of this Law.

use of hydroelectric potential.

Law 9.433/97 closes this list of examples with a clause of legislative openness, namely item V of article 12, which expressly refers to other uses that alter the regime, quantity or quality of the water in a body of water. As a result, it is possible to conclude that all uses that affect the regime, quantity and quality of water will be controlled by the Government through licensing, i.e. uses with the potential to damage water resources will be licensed. Among the uses with the potential to cause damage to water resources are, of course, those intended for economic activity in the broadest sense.

On the other hand, it is also true to say that uses that are not intended for economic activity are exempt from licensing, given their intrinsic relationship with the minimum existential requirement. In fact, the Water Law recognizes that certain uses should not be subject to licensing control because they are intended to meet the existential minimum.

Thus, recognizing that there is a right to the minimum conditions for a dignified human existence which cannot be the object of state intervention and which also requires positive state services, as has already been explained at length[272] , the Water Law subjects the following uses to the immunity regime: the use of water resources to satisfy the needs of small populations distributed in rural areas; derivations, abstractions and releases considered insignificant; accumulations of volumes of water considered insignificant.

Uses that have harmful potential are subject to licensing. However, uses intended to meet the minimum existential needs, which are not exploited by any economic sector, cannot be granted.

Thus, through the list in §1 of art. 12, the law seeks to safeguard the existential minimum, while the *caput of* the article discriminates against uses related to economic activity that can generate pollution, harmful alteration of the level of the water body, etc. Hence the

---

[272] TORRES, Ricardo Lobo. Treatise on constitutional financial and tax law - human rights and taxation: immunities and isonomy. ..., p 171.

need for these uses to be closely controlled by the State.

7.3. Water charges: tax nature.

In order to identify a certain fact qualified by a legal rule as establishing a tax, one has to look at the definition of tax and observe whether the fact legalized through the legal rule can be qualified as such. Heleno Taveira Torres' warning in this regard is timely: "If a type of 'public entry' does not fit into the respective concept of 'tax', by comparison, the immediate consequence is that the constitutional tax regime does not apply, because it does not fit into the respective concept of tax"[273] .

Without further debate on the definition of a tax, we will use the legal definition, with some doctrinal considerations, as a starting point. Art. 3 of the National Tax Code provides the legal definition of a tax, which is: "Art. 3 Tribute is any compulsory pecuniary payment, in currency or whose value can be expressed in it, which does not constitute a penalty for an unlawful act, established by law and collected through a fully binding administrative activity".

7.3.1. Obligation established by law or obligation *ex voluntate?*

Analyzing the nature of the obligation established by Law 9.433/97 in its article 20 is the starting point for affirming or denying the tax nature of the charge. First of all, it must be analyzed whether the obligation to pay a certain amount of money into the public coffers arises from the will of the parties or from the law. If the obligation arises from the will of the parties,

---

[273] TORRES, Heleno Taveira. The relationship ..., p.120-121.

and is a conventional figure *(obligatio ex voluntate),* the tax classification of the institute is definitively ruled out; however, if the obligation arises from the law *(obligatio ex lege)* it is possible that it is a tax, but this will be conditional on other requirements being met, such as whether or not the obligation arises from a lawful act. According to Geraldo Ataliba:

> If, on the other hand, the obligation arises independently of the will of the parties - or even against that will - by force of law, through the occurrence of a lawful legal event, then we are dealing with a tax, which is defined as a legal, pecuniary obligation, which is not a sanction for an unlawful act, in favor of a public person. There will be an obligation to compensate for damage if the fact from which the obligation arises is unlawful[274].

Therefore, if the tax rule refers to the creation of an obligation as a free consequence of the manifestation of a tax, it is not a tax obligation, it is not a tax. Nor is a tax obligation one which, although created by law, constitutes a penalty for an illegal act[275].

It is also worth mentioning the position of the Federal Supreme Court regarding the indemnity/compensation established through Law 7.990/1989 by virtue of art. 20, §1 of the Federal Constitution. The High Court held that the fact that the obligation to indemnify was instituted *ex lege* did not transform the figure outlined in that legal diploma into a tax[276]. In fact, it is compensation set by law. This goes to show that, in order to constitute a tax, the other elements of the legal definition must be present. In the case under analysis, the element relating to collection by a fully binding activity did not contribute to the definition of the figure, because, in fact, there is an accounting arrangement, which imposes the transfer.

According to Geraldo Ataliba: "In order for it to be a tax, the command 'pay money to the state' must be linked to the hypothesis 'if event x happens that is not illicit'"[277].

Water charges do not derive from a contractual link, since Law 9.433/97 itself creates

---

[274] ATALIBA, Geraldo. Hipotese de Incidencia Tributaria. 6 ed., 3ª tiragem, Sao Paulo: Malheiros, 2002, p. 37.
[275] Ibid., p. 57.
[276] RE 228.800, DJ 13/12/2002.
[277] ATALIBA, Geraldo. Hypothesis ..., p. 57.

the obligation for the taxpayer to pay the public coffers for uses subject to a grant (art. 20). The

obligation does not derive from a contract or agreement between the user and the State. The

rule, expressed in language that carries the obligatory deontic modal, determines that all use

subject to a grant will be charged for. Thus, the contract is ruled out as the source of the

obligation to pay for the use that can be granted. Therefore, it is possible that it is a tax.

Luciano Amaro believes that compulsory nature is not necessary to characterize a tax,

in the sense that it is a compulsory service, "because other legal services (employment, rent,

wages, etc.) are also compulsory, in the sense that the debtor does not perform them if he

wants to, but because he must (under penalty of being subject to judicial constriction).

Qualifying the (tax) payment as compulsory does not particularize or specify anything."[278] .

The compulsory nature of the tax is dependent on the fact that it has been instituted by

law. In this analysis, therefore, we consider the fact that the service is compulsory to be due to

the fact that it was instituted by law. Hence Luciano Amaro's assertion that

> We believe that the Code did not intend to say what it says (i.e. compulsory
> "payment"). It certainly meant to express that the obligation to pay (the tax) is
> compulsory (or forced), in the sense that this duty is created by force of law
> (obligation *ex lege),* and not by the will of the subjects of the legal relationship
> (obligation *ex voluntate).* In this sense, however, the expression is redundant, since
> the establishment of a tax by law is already an integral part of the concept of tax, and
> this circumstance should not be stated twice in the same definition.[279]

Although authors such as Leandro Paulsen point out that the distinctive feature of a tax

is that it is compulsory,

> there are pecuniary services provided for by law that do not constitute a tax because
> they lack, for example, such as financial compensation for the exploitation of mineral
> resources, which presupposes a decision by the private individual to exploit a public
> asset and pay the Union its share, or the so-called occupation tax on marine land, a
> kind of rent paid by the private individual for using a public asset in a private
> capacity (on the occupation tax and its nature, see note to art. 145, II, of the

---

[278] AMARO, Luciano. Brazilian Tax Law. 9. ed., Sao Paulo: Saraiva, 2003, p. 21.
[279] AMARO, Luciano. Tax Law ..., p. 21.

In this specific case, it was not the compulsory nature of the financial compensation that led the Federal Supreme Court to declare that the financial compensation established in Laws 7.990/89 and 8.001/90 was not a tax, but rather the fact that the other elements of the concept of a tax did not concur in the aforementioned case (not being a penalty for an illegal act and being levied by a fully binding activity).

It should also be noted that the case law of the Superior Court of Justice itself, in order to indicate, in the case of service charges, that the public service is compulsory, recalls the obligation in some legal diploma (see REsp 818649, DJ 02.05.2006 p. 273, cited in the previous item).

Therefore, it is possible to state that the charge fulfills the first requirement of the legal definition of a tax, which is that it is an obligation established by law and that it is compulsory.

7.3.2. Water charges: a penalty for an illegal act?

The essence of a tax cannot correspond to a penalty for practicing an illegal act. It is the duty of solidarity, in the sense that the community is co-responsible for the maintenance of the state and the provision of public services, which determines the establishment of the tax levy rule.

You don't pay tax because you have committed an illegal act, although you may have to pay it in abstraction from the fact that it has been committed, as in the case of paying income tax on income earned illegally (art. 118, inc. I of the National Tax Code).

---

[280] PAULSEN, Leandro. Tax Law: Constitution and Tax Code in the light of doctrine and case law. 7. ed. rev. atual. Porto Alegre: Livraria do Advogado: ESMAFE, 2005, p. 661.

<blockquote>
Tax is not a sanction for an illegal act and, therefore, the legislator cannot abstractly place the illegal act as the generator of the tax obligation or scale the amount due because of the illegality (e.g. setting a higher rate for income tax in relation to income from gambling). However, the underlying illegality is irrelevant. The acquisition of income and the promotion of the circulation of goods, for example, are, abstractly considered, lawful and taxable events. If the income was acquired illegally, if the goods could not be sold in the country, these are facts that go beyond the tax issue, they are underlying illicitnesses that do not rule out taxation[281] .
</blockquote>

It is forbidden in our legal system to use a tax for the purpose of penalizing unlawfulness, and it is therefore inadmissible to increase the rate or calculation basis of a tax with a view to unlawfulness.

Having said that, we will now analyze water charges.

A simple analysis of art. 49 et seq. of Law 9.433/97 is enough to show that charging is not a sanction for an illegal act. These provisions provide for the imposition of a financial penalty, in addition to other sanctions, for non-compliance with water legislation[282] . It should be noted that the legislator expressly and topographically separated what he considered to be an instrument for implementing the National Water Resources Policy (collection - art. 19 et seq.) and what he considered to be a pecuniary penalty resulting from non-compliance with the legislation, or rather, the imposition of a sanction for an illegal act (fine - art. 49).

There is also no doubt that the purpose of charging is to gradually raise collective awareness of the importance of rationalizing the use of water and to raise funds to finance activities to recover and preserve water resources (art. 19). The purpose of the charge reveals

---

[281] PAULSEN, Leandro. Direito Tributario..., p. 664. In the same vein, the STF has already ruled (1ª T., unanimous, HC 77.530, rel. Min. Sepulveda Pertence, Aug/1999): EMENTA: Tax evasion of profits from criminal activity: "non olet". Drugs: drug trafficking, involving organized commercial companies, with large profits withheld from the regular accounting of the companies and withheld from income declarations: characterization, in theory, of the crime of tax evasion, entailing the jurisdiction of the Federal Court and attracting, by connection, the trafficking of narcotics: irrelevance of the illicit origin, even when criminal, of the income withheld from taxation. The tax exemption of the economic results of a criminal act - before being a corollary of the principle of morality - constitutes a violation of the principle of fiscal isonomy, of manifest ethical inspiration.

[282] Art. 50 - For infringement of any legal or regulatory provision relating to the execution of hydraulic works and services, derivation or use of water resources in the domain or administration of the Union, or for failure to comply with requests made, the infringer, at the discretion of the competent authority, shall be subject to the following penalties, regardless of their order of listing: II - a simple or daily fine, proportional to the seriousness of the infringement, from R$ 100.00 (one hundred reais) to R$ 10.000.00 (ten thousand reais).

that the aim behind its creation was not to penalize individuals for committing an illegal act, but rather to discourage activities that pollute water resources, avoiding the hydro-environmental impacts shared by all water bodies.

Thus, charging for water is not the consequence of an illegal act, nor is it intended to penalize an individual for committing an illegal act; on the contrary, the aim of the extra-fiscal tax, which is conveyed through charging, is precisely to encourage conduct that preserves the environment and, specifically, water. Charging has a prohibitive extra-fiscal purpose, which cannot be conceived as the imposition of a penalty for an illegal act. Hugo de Brito Machado warns that

> the prohibitive extrafiscal tax, as we have already said and as we all know, has the same objective as a penalty, in other words, it has the same objective as a sanction, in other words, it aims to discourage certain conduct. Therefore, on an axiological level, the distinction is impossible. The penalty, as we have seen, presupposes an unlawful act. It is a consequence of not providing services. The prohibitive extrafiscal tax, on the other hand, has no illicit act in its hypothesis of incidence[283] .

Therefore, although extrafiscal taxation has an axiological motivation similar to that of a sanction, it does not allow sanctions and prohibitive extrafiscal taxation to be confused, because a sanction is an imputation for non-compliance with a legally imposed duty; extrafiscal tax obligation has nothing to do with illegality, the hypothesis of incidence is not formed by an illicit fact, on the contrary, the hypothesis of incidence of this type of tax is a licit fact, but that the State, through taxation, wants to discourage from occurring, as determined by Arthur Pigou.

Thus, the water charge is another element of the concept of a tax: it is not a penalty for an illegal act.

---

[283] MACHADO, Hugo de Brito. The Concept of Tribute in Brazilian Law. Rio de Janeiro: Forense, 1987, p. 39.

7.3.3. Water charges: expressed in currency or the value of which can be expressed in currency.

This aspect does not give rise to major problems, since the water charge will necessarily be expressed in monetary terms (see the section on the value of water resources), which will revert to the public coffers in order to finance studies, programs, projects and works included in the Water Resources Plans and to pay, limited to 7.5% of the amounts collected, for the implementation and administrative costs of the bodies and entities that make up the National Water Resources Management System.

Furthermore, the aim of quantifying the value of water is at the heart of the National Water Policy itself, which is based on the economic valuation of water (art. 1, inc. II, of Law 9.433/97).

7.3.4. Charging for water: required through a fully binding administrative activity.

This aspect is extremely important for characterizing a given obligation as a tax obligation. Having verified that the water charge is a compulsory obligation, established by law, which does not constitute a penalty for an unlawful act and is expressed in currency or the value of which can be expressed in currency, in order to legally characterize the charge as a tax it remains to be analyzed whether it is collected through a fully binding activity.

Hugo de Brito Machado warns that administrators prefer to use the expression "binding power" instead of "binding activity".

The activity of the Administration can be arbitrary, binding or discretionary, according to the vast majority of Administrative Law textbooks. Binding activities are those in which the administrative authority does not have the freedom to judge whether it is advisable and appropriate to act. The law would establish an end to be achieved, the form to be observed and the authority's competence to act, as well as setting the time to act and the content of the activity itself. Therefore, a binding activity would leave no room for discretion on the part of the authority, which would be entirely bound by the legal command[284].

Today we recognize measures that, by using less precise normative and/or evaluative concepts, remove a certain margin of binding administrative action. This is because the terms themselves impose an effort on the interpreter to fill in their meaning.

Thus, this binding of the administrative agent is a question of degree of intensity, because "the 'binding' act does not have a different nature from the 'discretionary' act, the difference in the degree of freedom of decision granted by the legislator being quantitative, but not qualitative. The administrative decision oscillates between the poles of full binding and full discretion"[285]. It is the mandatory density of the linguistic terms used that will determine the binding nature of the public administrator[286].

In tax law, the binding nature of the administrative activity of establishing the tax credit is at its highest. Hugo de Brito Machado, despite recognizing the above distinction, makes a good point:

> When the CTN says that the tax must be collected through a fully binding administrative activity, it means that the administrative authority cannot use its personal, subjective judgment to fill in the field of indeterminate rules, seeking to achieve the purpose of the law in each case. The law must be detailed, rigorously and objectively outlining the prerequisites for acts and their content. It must describe the taxable event, the calculation basis, the rate, the deadline for payment, the subjects of the tax relationship and everything else. Nothing is left to the discretion of the administrative authority in each case. When the law contains indeterminacies, these must be filled in normatively, in other words, by issuing a normative act, applicable to all those who find themselves in the situation hypothetically envisaged therein. Thus, the activity of determining and collecting the tax will always be linked to a

---

[284] MACHADO, Hugo de Brito. The Concept ..., p. 70.
[285] KRELL, Andreas J.. Discretion..., p. 22.
[286] Ibid., p. 23.

norm[287] .

It must be recognized that the hypothesis of incidence may contain undetermined concepts, but this does not give the public agent the option of not constituting the tax credit.

> In fact, the vagueness or indeterminacy of the concepts contained in the rule does not confer discretionary power on the holder of the competence it assigns. It does leave a certain margin of freedom in the exercise of that competence, but this freedom is not to be confused with that which characterizes discretion. The freedom arising from the vagueness or indeterminacy of concepts is not attributed to a particular authority, but a freedom that belongs to anyone who has to apply the rule. When the authority, in exercising the competence conferred by the rule in which vague or indeterminate concepts reside, interprets the concept, giving it a certain content, it is applying the rule with the meaning that in its view is correct. His understanding can be altered by another authority that has the power to exercise control over legality[288] .

The power to charge for water resources was given to the authority competent to grant the use of water resources. The Union, through Law 9.433/97, delegated to the states the power to collect directly or through the Water Agencies the resources arising from charging in the hydrographic basins located exclusively in their territories (art. 44, inc. III). The resources collected in the hydrographic basins of diffuse ownership included among the assets of the Union will be collected by the National Water Agency (art. 4, inc. VIII and IX of Law 9.984/2000).

In this respect, it is important to remember the difference between tax competence and tax capacity. In the precise words of Hugo de Brito Machado:

> The power to tax is attributed by the Constitution to a state entity with legislative power. It is exercised through the enactment of a law. Tax capacity, on the other hand, is attributed by the Constitution, or by a law, to a state entity not necessarily endowed with legislative power. It is exercised through administrative acts.
> The state entity endowed with legislative competence may also have tax capacity. By issuing a law, it exercises its competence, and by carrying out administrative acts, its

---

[287] MACHADO, Hugo de Brito. Curso de Direito Tributario. 24ª ed., rev., atual. e ampl., Sao Paulo: Malheiros, 2004, p. 70.
[288] MACHADO, Hugo de Brito. Course..., p. 70.

tax capacity[289] .

It should be remembered that it was established a long time ago that the power to legislate on water lies with the Union, and that the power to create the national water resources management system and its respective instruments lies with the Union. The understanding was also established that the ownership of water resources, affirmed in the Constitution, is not by way of *dominus,* but only by way of manager of the environmental asset located in its territory, and that the Public Power is not the owner of the water, because it is a diffuse asset. Therefore, the old rhetorical discourse that the Public Power can institute remuneration for the use of its assets, through public procurement, in matters of environmental assets, does not apply, because strictly speaking the asset is diffuse, belonging to everyone and to the Public Power.

Well then, if the Union is the constitutionally competent entity to establish public water policies, to manage the national water system and to legislate on water, it is the legislative power of this entity that can create a tax on water. And so it did when it created the figure of the levy, established in art. 19 et seq. of the Water Law, i.e. the levy is created by the Union and the taxing power to collect the resources is delegated to the states, which can hand it over to the Water Agencies.

It is already well-established that the entity competent to create the tax can delegate the taxing power to other entities. It is enough to note that social security contributions are collected by an autarchy (INSS) and the environmental control and inspection fee is collected by an autarchy (IBAMA)[290] , whereas, in these cases, the competence to institute the tax lies with the Union.

In the case of river basins that are the "domain" of the Union, the charge is collected by

---

[289] Ibid., p. 70.
[290] According to article 17-Q of Law 6.938/81, IBAMA can pass on, as Law 9.433/97 did, part of the revenue collected from the environmental control and inspection fee.

122

an autarchy, the ANA, and in river basins that are the "domain" of the states, the charge is collected directly by the states or by the Water Agencies that they set up (Art. 7 of the CTN).

Therefore, there is no doubt that the public official who is asked to grant a water concession has no other duty than to collect the amount of the charge from the public coffers, which is the last requirement to characterize the water charge as a tax.

7.4. Water charges: a tax, its species and the need to situate the issue constitutionally.

The charge fits perfectly into the legal concept of Article 3 of the CTN and is therefore a tax. What kind? There are different doctrines on tax species. For some, there is a dichotomous division of tax species[291] , which would be taxes (which would include all taxes not linked to state action) and fees (which would include all taxes linked to state action). In the latter case, it doesn't matter whether the triggering event is a service, work or act of police power or economic intervention, and the specific state action derived from the payment of the tax is enough to classify it as a fee.

There are those who belong to the trichotomous school, according to which there are three types of tax: taxes, fees and improvement contributions[292] . For them, parafiscal contributions and compulsory loans are taxes or fees[293] . A variation on the tripartite division is that of Geraldo Ataliba[294] , who believes that there are taxes, fees and contributions (divided

---

[291] The dichotomous school takes into account the tax base in particular. "Taxes are instituted and then levied because a fact on the part of the taxpayer, an indicator of economic capacity, independently of any state action in relation to it, is taken as the taxable event or, on the contrary, because a specific, special state action in relation to the taxpayer is chosen as the taxable event". (COELHO, Sacha Calmon Navarro. Course in Brazilian Tax Law. Rio de Janeiro: Forense, 2001, p. 398).

[292] The tax base performs both the function of quantifying the amount payable and the veritative function, i.e. confirming or disconfirming the specific legal nature of the tax species. (COELHO, Sacha Calmon Navarro. Course in Brazilian Tax Law. Rio de Janeiro: Forense, 2001, p. 399).

[293] COELHO, Sacha Calmon Navarro. Course ..., p. 399.

[294] ATALIBA, Geraldo. Hypothesis ..., pp. 146-147.

into two species: improvement contributions and special contributions) .[295]

Others divide taxes into four types: taxes, fees, improvement contributions and special contributions. Finally, there are those authors, including the pacific jurisprudence of the Federal Supreme Court[296] , who use the pentapartite division of tax species, namely taxes, fees, improvement contributions, special contributions or art. 149 contributions and compulsory loans.

We have adopted Geraldo Ataliba's division here, according to which taxes are of three types: taxes, fees and contributions. The distinction between binding taxes (fees and contributions) and non-binding taxes (taxes) serves to differentiate tax from both fees and contributions.

The difference between taxes and contributions, according to Geraldo Ataliba, lies in the way in which state action refers to the obligor. The hypothesis of the levy would be a state action directly related to the obligor, while the hypothesis of the contribution is an activity indirectly related to the obligor (state action obliquely linked to the taxpayer)[297] . According to Geraldo Ataliba:

> In a fee, h.i. is the state providing a service, issuing a certificate, carrying out an activity aimed at culminating in giving or maintaining a license, permit, etc., which is linked to someone who is placed by law in the position of taxable person.
>
> From this it can be seen that, in order for a tax to be established, it is enough for the law to provide for state action that is referable to someone (who can be placed as the taxable person). This tax will be born with referability (at the moment when the state action refers concretely to something).
>
> In the case of contributions, on the other hand, state action is not enough. There is only a contribution when, between the state's action and the obliged party, the law places an intermediary term, which establishes the referability between the action itself and the obliged party. Hence the distinction between a fee and a contribution is based on the (direct or indirect) nature of the reference between the action and the obliged party.

---

[295] For Geraldo Ataliba, the use of the criterion that separates taxes into binding and non-binding is useful, which is why he claims that fees and contributions are different from taxes because the former refer to a specific state action and the latter do not refer to a specific state action.

[296] RE 138.284, RE 146.733 and ADC 1/DF.

[297] ATALIBA, Geraldo. Hypothesis ..., p. 147.

> In the case of a contribution, there is a circumstance, an intermediary fact, between the action and the obligor. It is through this fact or circumstance that referability is established between the state action and the obligor, which leads us to recognize that this referability is mediated, in contrast to what happens in the tax.
>
> In the case of a contribution, you either have a state action that produces an effect, which (effect) is connected to someone else (who is, by law, placed in the position of taxable person), or, on the contrary, you have a person (who will ultimately be a taxable person) who carries out an activity, or causes a situation that requires, demands, provokes or triggers a state action. activity, or causes a situation that requires, demands, provokes or triggers state action[298] .

This criterion of mediated or immediate referability between the taxable person and the state's action is the major difference between a binding tax such as a fee and a binding tax such as a contribution.

Still on the subject of tax types, it is necessary to establish some constitutional requirements for their creation. For the creation of certain taxes, the Constitution demands greater rigors in the legislative process. This is the case of taxes created through residual competence and social contributions whose legal fact is not provided for in the sections of art. 195 of the Charter of the Republic. The other types of tax will be created by ordinary law.

It should be noted that the levy was instituted by ordinary law. Thus, if the levy were a tax created through residual competence (art. 154, inc. I of the Federal Constitution) or a social contribution not provided for in the sections of art. 195, it would be unconstitutional, because it would have been created through an ordinary law and not a complementary law as required by the Charter of the Republic. However, the levy is not a residual tax (non-binding tax), because its revenue is earmarked for a specific purpose. Nor is it a social contribution, because its specific purpose is not to finance social security.

It should be noted that it is understood that the establishment of a contribution to intervene in the economic domain does not require a complementary law[299] . In fact, the reference that art. 149 of the Constitution makes to art. 146, inc. III refers to the discipline

---

Creation. *In:* Contribution of intervention in the economic domain and related figures. Coordinator Marco Aurelio Greco. Sao Paulo Dialetica, 2001, p. 28.

provided for in the CTN, but not to the indispensability of a prior complementary law to institute it.

It is possible, as stated above, to rule out from the outset that the levy does not fall under the legal regime of taxes, because it is undeniable, from the very wording of the law, that it is linked to the purpose, as has already been exhaustively explained, of preserving and conserving water bodies from pollution and predatory activity that reduces their quality and quantity. Therefore, the charge can be a fee or a contribution.

Furthermore, it is possible to rule out the classification of water charges as an improvement contribution, because the increase has no reference to a public work. Nor is it an exaggeration intended to finance social security or a professional category.

From the above, it remains to analyze the fees (service and police) and the contributions for intervention in the economic domain to see which regime the water charge best fits into.

7.4.1. Service charge and police charge *versus* economic intervention contribution.

The fee, as we have seen, is a tax linked to a state action directly related to the taxpayer, which the Constitution states in art. 145 can be the exercise of police power or the actual or potential use of a specific and divisible public service. Thus, doctrine usually subdivides it into service fees and police fees.

In the case of taxes, the taxable event has to be an occurrence related to the use, provocation or provision of the service or activity of the State: invoking the functioning of the justice system, regularizing measuring and weighing instruments, etc. That's why Geraldo

Ataliba concludes that you can't demand a fee for a mail service that you didn't use, or a fee for an inspection that you didn't do[300] . Therefore, only those who use the public service or receive the "police" act can be subject to a tax.

The tax base, the material aspect of the hypothesis of incidence, of service charges will generally be the cost of the service provided directly to taxpayers. The service must be specific (provision of material utility, individually enjoyable by the administered, under public law) and divisible (or rather, it must be possible to separate units of use for individual enjoyment by the administered).

Law 9.433/97 does not establish a service charge, because the activity specified there for taxation is the preservation of the hydric environment from pollution and predatory activities, with a view to guaranteeing the right to access to water for all, in sufficient quality and quantity for present and future generations, which is why it is the permitted uses that will be charged (art. 20[301]), because, as we have seen, the grant "aims to ensure the quantitative and qualitative control of water uses and the effective exercise of rights of access to water" (art. 11). Therefore, the state activity provided with the grant and charge is the preservation of water bodies, as can also be seen in the content of art. 19 and art. 22 of Law 9.433/97, *in litteris:*

> Art. 19: Charging for the use of water resources aims to:
> I - recognize water as an economic asset and give users an indication of its real value;
> II - encourage the rational use of water;
> III - obtain financial resources to finance the programs and interventions included in the water resources plans.
> IV - its variation regime and the flsico-chemical, biological and toxicity characteristics of the tributary.
>
> Art. 22: The amounts collected from charging for the use of water resources shall be applied as a priority in the hydrographic basin in which they were generated and will be used:

---

[300] ATALIBA, Geraldo. Hypothesis ..., p. 156.
[301] Art. 20: Charges will be levied for the use of water resources subject to granting, under the terms of art. 12 of this Law.

<blockquote>
I - in the financing of studies, programs, projects and works included in the Water Resources Plans;

II - in the payment of implementation and administrative costs of the bodies and entities that make up the National Water Resources Management System.
</blockquote>

So, one wonders: is there a state service directly linked to the taxpayer? Clearly not, because these activities to preserve and conserve the environment, specifically water bodies, as a right of all (in the wording of art. 225 of the Charter of the Republic), only mediate the specific interests of the individual. Therefore, it is not a specific and divisible public service.

One might ask: isn't the exercise of the state's police power actually described in the hypothesis of incidence?

Paulo Roberto Lyrio Pimenta highlights some differences between intervention contributions and police fees[302] , found in the material criteria of the hypothesis of incidence and the tax base. The material criterion for a police tax is the effective exercise of police power; in the case of an economic intervention contribution, the material criterion can be any fact that falls within the scope of the Union's material competence. The taxable base for police fees is the cost of inspection, while the intervention contribution measures "a fact unrelated to any activity of the state, since the intervention does not constitute the materiality of the exaction"[303] .

The author explains that the Constitution did not establish, as it did for taxes, fees and improvement contributions, the material criterion that legitimizes the establishment of an intervention contribution, but rather used the technique of finalist validation[304] , or rather its

---

[302] PIMENTA, Paulo Roberto Lyrio. Constitutional profile of economic intervention contributions. *In:* Contribution of intervention in the economic domain and related figures. Coordinator Marco Aurdlio Greco. Sao Paulo Dialdtica, 2001, p. 171.

[303] Ibid., p. 171.

[304] In the finalist validation technique, the ends are defined in the Federal Constitution itself, and it is up to the legislator to choose the most appropriate means to achieve the stated ends. (PIMENTA, Paulo Roberto Lyrio. Contributions for Intervention in the Economic Domain. Sao Paulo: Dialdtica, 2002, p.16-17)

purpose, which will constitutionally legitimize the intervention contribution[305] . The purposes must be constitutionally qualified[306] , which are those provided for in articles 173 and 174 of the Constitution of the Republic. Heleno Taveira Torres teaches this:

> Police power and state control, normally carried out through acts of inspection. This requires a public body to be created and functioning, so that a "fee" can be charged for effective state action. Contribution for Intervention in the Economic Domain, on the other hand, can only be instituted in cases where it is in the interest of promoting a certain economic segment (stimulus) or discouraging action in a certain economic domain, through the collection itself (discouragement). It therefore has nothing to do with police power, as it is based on the foundations of the interventionist state[307] .

Marco Aurdlio Greco also weighs in:

> On the other hand, if the fields of activity are configured as belonging to the so-called economic activity, over which the Public Power can exercise police power (activity of controlling the adequacy of the behavior of private individuals to the dictates of the law), this does not mean that there is an impediment to the creation of an intervention contribution. In other words, the mere fact that there is a type of Union activity does not prevent the creation of the contribution. There will be an impediment if the field of activity taken as a reference for the requirement is a public service. Police power, although it is a type of state activity, is supposed to cover the conduct of private individuals in the non-public sphere, often in the field of economic activity. In short, while the field of service excludes the intervention contribution, the field of police power is compatible with it, which means that the same sector of economic activity can be subject to both fees for the exercise of police power and the contribution for intervention in the economic domain, since both have a constitutional profile, foundation and assumption that are compatible, and not mutually exclusive.[308]

Therefore, it is not possible to classify the water charge as a police fee, because in the material aspect of the hypothesis of incidence there is no specific duty to supervise, the exaction created by Law 9.433/97 is closer to an intervention contribution, because it is the purposes pursued and expressed in Law 9.433/97 that constitutionally legitimize the

---

[305] Ibid., p.59.
[306] Cf. the doctrine of Geraldo Ataliba, Marco Aurelio Greco, Roque Antonio Carraza, Misabel Derzi, among others.
[307] TORRES, Heleno Taveira. The relationship ..., p.144.
[308] GRECO, Marco Aurelio. Contribution ..., p. 15.

contribution. In fact, the purpose of charging for water is to discourage economic activities that are harmful to the quantity and quality of water resources. Take a look at the objective set out in art. 19 of Law 9.433/97.

The analysis of the tax base for water charges also bears no relation to the cost of the inspection activity; on the contrary, the calculation base is the volume abstracted or emitted into the water body (art. 21). In the case of water charges, the police power is just one way of achieving the aim set out in art. 174[309] .

Paulo Roberto Lyrio Pimenta points out other aspects that serve to distinguish a tax from an intervention contribution:

> In the case of a police tax, the state's action is provoked by the taxpayer, while in the case of an interventional contribution it can be provoking or provoked. In the case of fees, the police power is directed at a specific subject, while in the case of contributions it is aimed at a group. In police taxes, validation is causal. The tax is paid "because" the police power has been exercised. In the case of intervention contributions, the validation is final. Therefore, the tax is collected "so that" the intervention takes place through the exercise of police power. The fee is a reward for the efforts made by the public authority to carry out the act of policing, while contributions may or may not be intended to cover the cost of a state activity. In the case of fees, the action of the Administration consists of an individual and concrete act. In the case of contributions, it may consist of issuing general rules or carrying out concrete acts. The handing over of money is part of the antecedent of the rule imposing police fees. In the case of contributions, it is part of the consequent or antecedent. The reference to state action is direct in the case of fees and indirect in the case of contributions. The public interest in fees is not necessarily economic, while in contributions it is essential. In fees, the power to police is qualified negatively, i.e. the content is given by exclusion: everything that does not fall within the scope of art. 174 can represent the materiality of fees. In intervention contributions, the power to police is positively qualified by art. 174, and has specific content[310]

After this brief explanation, *it is* possible to state that the water charge is not a service charge, nor is it a police charge. As anticipated, by denying that it is a fee, the water charge is a contribution, of the type of intervention in the economic domain. Heleno Taveira Torres had already seen that:

---

309 PIMENTA, Paulo Roberto Lyrio. Contribuigoes ..., p.51.
310 PIMENTA, Paulo Roberto Lyrio. Profile..., p.p. 171-172.

is found in Law 9.433, of 8.1.1997, which establishes the policy of water resources, when the "granting of rights to use water resources" was created, provided for in art. 19 of that law, which we understand as a typical type of CIDE, despite the irregularities presented, such as the lack of definition of the rates, which was left to ANA Resolutions, in direct affront to the principle of legality[311] .

7.4.2. Legal destination of revenue.

Contributions for intervention in the economic domain are instituted to achieve certain constitutionally qualified purposes[312] . The 1988 Constitution delimited the modalities and assumptions of intervention in the economic domain, in such a way as to bind the purpose to a certain constitutional framework. Another essential characteristic follows from this: the proceeds must necessarily be used for the purpose for which the tax was created .[313]

An essential characteristic, according to an authoritative sector of the doctrine, is that the purpose became, with the 1988 Constitution, a criterion capable of differentiating the tax species[314] . In this sense, the doctrine warns that the purpose that characterizes the contribution and authorizes its collection cannot be confused with the actual destination of the resources, in the world of facts for that purpose. Thus, the legal destination or purpose would constitute the constitutional validation circle for some types of tax. It follows that the power to tax derives from the purposes to be pursued[315] .

According to Leandro Paulsen, art. 4 of the CTN does not apply to the intervention contribution, because the provision uses the concept of legal destination and not constitutional destination.

---

[311] TORRES, Heleno Taveira. The relationship ..., p. 108.
[312] PIMENTA, Paulo Roberto Lyrio. Contributions ..., p. 17
[313] Ibid., p. 18.
[314] In agreement with this view: Leandro Paulsen, Hugo de Brito Machado, Luis Eduardo Schoueri, Paulo Roberto Lyrio Pimenta.
[315] PAULSEN, Leandro. Law..., p.668.

Through charging, Law 9.433/97 seeks to preserve and protect water resources in sufficient quality and quantity for present and future generations, preventing predatory uses capable of affecting the water regime, thus imposing limitations on economic activity, so that both abstractions, derivations and effluent emissions into water bodies do not harm the environment (arts. 11, 19, 20, 22 of Law 9.433/97, already exhaustively cited)[316].

An environmental tax cannot be one that simply serves to form a "fund" for this purpose. As Pedro Herrera points out, a tax does not become an environmental tax simply because its proceeds are earmarked for environmental protection[317]. Therefore, the fact that the revenue collected is earmarked for a "fund" is not enough to confer constitutional validation, since the collection must be used to fulfill the constitutional purpose.

7.5. *Identification of the aspects that characterize water charging.*

The levy established by Law 9.433/97, when analyzed in the light of tax law theory, must be broken down into its various aspects - Geraldo Ataliba rejects the use of the term element, as he considers that both the hypothesis of incidence and the taxable event are one and the same[318]. Taking Paulo de Barros Carvalho's doctrine into account, this work specifies the set of criteria capable of identifying the lawful fact contained in the hypothesis of incidence (material, temporal and spatial criteria) and the set of criteria capable of identifying a legal

---

[316] It must be recognized, however, that despite the fact that linkage is a valid criterion, the funds collected from economic intervention contributions have not always been used for the legally prescribed purpose. Today, despite the fact that water charges are already being implemented, even without meeting, in our opinion, all the constitutional and legal requirements, the contigion and detour of the funds collected is already taking place, as Maria Luiza Wernek dos Santos informs us, despite the fact that "they have already been collected since August 2000 - generating amounts in the order of R$88 million up to 2002, R$96 million in 2004 and an estimated R$107.68 million in 2005 - they have been systematically cut back by the Executive Branch, 77.7% in 2004, and for this year, the LDO already foresees a further 80% cutback". (On the application of the resources earned from charging for water use. The illegitimacy of its contingency. The normative competence of the CNRH and the ANA. *In:* Administrative Law - Studies in honor of Diogo de Figueiredo Moreira Neto. Coord. Fabio Medina Osorio e Marcos Juruena Villela Souto, Rio de Janeiro: Lumen Juris, 2006, p. 956).
[317] TORRES, Heleno Taveira. The relationship ..., p. 109.
[318] ATALIBA, Geraldo. Hypothesis ..., p. 77.

relationship in which the active subject is the State; the taxable person is a natural or legal person; and the object, a payment of a pecuniary nature, contained in the consequent of the rule (personal and quantitative criteria, the latter including the calculation basis and rate)[319].

7.5.1. Material criteria.

As stated above, the Major Text did not provide, as it did with other taxes, for the material criterion of the hypothesis of incidence. In the case of economic intervention taxes, the constituent legislator adopted the technique of finalist validation, through which the constitutionally established purpose will give validity to the exaggeration.

Any fact with an economic content can be included as a material criterion, as long as the Union does not invade the tax field that the Major Law has reserved for other political entities. Rather, it must strictly observe the principle of the reservation of tax powers, choosing as the hypothesis of incidence the facts that the Constitution has allowed to be taxed[320].

Roque Antonio Carrazza informs us, inspired by Mizabel Derzi, that "intervention in the economic domain may take place to defend the consumer, to preserve the environment, to guarantee the participation of States, Municipalities and the Federal District in the result of the exploitation, in their respective territories, of mineral resources, etc."[321].

The materiality of the hypothesis lies in the need to intervene in economic activity in such a way that the quality and quantity of water resources are preserved. It should be noted that uses aimed at ensuring the minimum existential level are not subject to granting and, consequently, charging. This is what Ricardo Lobo Torres developed as the immunity of the

---

[319] CARVALHO, Paulo de Barros. Teoria da norma tributaria. Sao Paulo: Max Limonad, 1998, p. 99 et seq.
[320] CARRAZA, Roque Antonio. Course in Constitutional Tax Law. 22ª ed. Sao Paulo: Malheiros Editores, 2006, p. 563.
[321] CARRAZA, Roque Antonio. Course ..., p. 563.

existential minimum.

It should be emphasized that it is the Union's exclusive competence to create the economic domain contribution by means of an ordinary law. It has also been established that it is the Union's responsibility to ensure the protection of water resources, unifying national policy, creating all the instruments capable of preventing the predatory use of water and, above all, legislating privately in this field. Therefore, in the field of water, above any other environmental issue that could lead to a discussion about competing competences, the only entity entitled to tax is the Union.

7.5.2. Spatial criteria.

The spatial aspect aims to indicate the circumstances of place, contained in the hypothesis of incidence, which are relevant to the configuration of the taxable event. It must be ascertained whether the taxable event occurred within the territorial ambit in which the law is valid.

On the other hand, the law can emphasize or highlight the spatial aspect of the hypothesis of incidence, adding to this geographic conditioning a specific fact of place, considered decisive for the very configuration of the taxable events[322] .

Law 9.433/97 reveals throughout its design the adoption of a special determining circle, which will also be reflected in the configuration of the taxable event, namely the hydrographic basin (see arts. 1, inc. V, 37 and others). This circle will have an impact on the uses that can be granted. In fact, the competence prescribed in art. 38, inc. V states that the Basin Committee can point out accumulations, derivations, abstractions and releases that it considers to be of little significance in order to exempt them from licensing. By exempting the

---

[322] ATALIBA, Geraldo. Hypothesis ..., p. 105.

grant, the Committee ends up interfering in the charge, since it will be removing that use from the hypothesis of incidence.

7.5.3. Time criterion.

Every hypothesis of incidence explicitly or implicitly contains the moment at which the taxable event is considered to have occurred, to have been consummated. Geraldo Ataliba warns that the hypothesis of incidence is usually implicit[323] . The legislator may omit to designate the moment at which the taxable event is deemed to have been consummated, if he does so "he will be implicitly providing that the moment to be considered is the one at which the material fact described occurs (happens)"[324] .

By determining the time at which the taxable event will be considered to have occurred, the moment at which the tax obligation arises is indicated, as well as which rule will govern the specific case.

Traditional doctrine uses the temporal aspect to classify taxable events, in terms of structure into simple and complex and, in terms of process, into complex, instantaneous and continuous. Paulo de Barros Carvalho points out the uselessness of the first classification, since what matters to the Law are not the moments that precede the birth of the tax obligation, but the result on which the precept will fall, triggering legal effects. Also with regard to the tripartite classification, the author states that this ignores the fact that the incidence of tax law is automatic, because

For this to be possible, we would have to be able to conceive of an event happening

---

[323] Ibid., p. 94.
[324] Ibid., p. 94.

Following a similar line of thought, we have adopted the classification proposed by the aforementioned professor, which would be 1) hypotheses of incidence that provide for an exact moment for the taxable event to occur and 2) hypotheses of incidence that do not allude to the moment when the taxable event must occur.

With these considerations in mind, we will now analyze the collection in terms of time. Article 20 of Law 9.433/97 is the first reference point for determining when the taxable event will be considered to have occurred. This article states: "Charges will be levied for the use of water resources subject to a grant, under the terms of art. 12 of this Law".

The provision does not set the exact moment from which the taxable event will be considered to have occurred, but it does impose a logical limitation that prevents the taxable event from occurring before the grant. Indeed, if only those uses that can be granted are charged, it is not possible to charge if the competent authority does not verify that the grant is feasible. Thus, the taxable event cannot be considered to have occurred until the granting process has been processed and a decision has been made as to whether it is feasible to claim for the derivation, abstraction and extraction of water or the discharge of sewage and other liquid or gaseous waste.

Article 21 of Law 9.433/97 gives another indication of when the taxable event should be considered to have occurred. It states that:

Art. 21: When setting the amounts to be charged for the use of water resources, the following must be observed, among others:
I - in the derivations, abstractions and extractions of water, the volume withdrawn and its rate of change;

---

[325] CARVALHO, Paulo de Barros. Tax Law Course. 14. ed. rev. and updated, Sao Paulo: Saraiva, 2002.

> II - when sewage and other liquid or gaseous waste is discharged, the volume discharged and its rate of change, as well as the physical-chemical, biological and toxic characteristics of the effluent.

Thus, the taxable event for charging should be considered to have occurred after the grant, when the derivation, abstraction, extraction or emission of effluents into water bodies begins. The wording of art. 21[326] makes it possible to construct the rule that dictates when the taxable event occurs, insofar as the amounts will be "fixed for derivations, abstractions, extractions or effluent emissions", i.e. after the grant and at the start of these activities.

7.5.4. Quantitative criteria

7.5.4.1 Tax base or calculation basis.

The calculation basis[327] is a dimensional perspective of the material aspect of the hypothesis of incidence.

When the contribution to intervene in the economic domain is required in order to achieve a purpose, the tax base can be calculated using volume, number of units, *per capita* values, etc. The legislator chose to establish the calculation basis on the basis of the volume captured, derived, extracted or emitted (art. 21[328]). This aspect is not controversial given the wording of the article in question.

---

[326] This statement informs not only the time credit but also the calculation basis.

[327] The terms 'base of calculation' and 'taxable base' will be used interchangeably, despite the doctrinal considerations regarding the indiscriminate use of these terms. For Geraldo Ataliba, the term 'taxable base' should be used, as not every tax would need to be calculated, and for Paulo de Barros Carvalho, the term 'taxable base' is criticized, using the term 'base of calculation'. (CARVALHO, Paulo de Barros. Direito Tributario: fundamentos juridicos da incidencia. 2.ed. rev., Sao Paulo: Saraiva, 1999, p. 170-171).

[328] Art. 21: When setting the amounts to be charged for the use of water resources, the following must be taken into account, among others: I - in water derivations, abstractions and extractions, the volume withdrawn and its variation; II - in sewage and other liquid or gaseous waste releases, the volume released and its variation and the physical-chemical, biological and toxicity characteristics of the tributary.

7.5.4.2. Rate.

Law 9.433/97 does not expressly define the amount to be charged. The Basin Committee is given the power to suggest, on the basis of studies carried out by the basin agencies[329] , the amounts to be charged (art. 38, VI[330]), in express reference to setting the rate.

The lack of legal designation of the rate can be seen as an affront to the principle of legal reserve.

> There is a certain type of tax that has no rate, as it is levied on a fixed amount previously determined by law. This is the case with some fees, where there is no relationship between the provision of the public service and the value of the benefit to the taxpayer, and some taxes on juridical acts or on the assumption "constituted by the simple fact of the existence of a person subject to the financial power of the public entity, as was the case with the tax on celibacy". It would be unfair and deeply discriminatory, however, to levy a flat-rate tax when there is a measurable basis for calculation, capable of supporting the levying of proportional or progressive rates. It would therefore be unconstitutional to levy proportional IPTU and ITBI through fixed amounts previously established by law[331] .

There are respectable scholars who opine on the possibility of a flat-rate tax, including Sacha Calmon, Ives Gandra Martins, Misabel Derzi, Luciano Amaro[332] . However, this is not the majority doctrine. In this case, it is worth noting that, even if it is possible to defend the flat tax, Law 9.433/97 itself is silent on this point and can therefore be considered unconstitutional.

Indeed, the fact that there is no rate does not mean that the contribution in kind is a fixed tax. This rate has been set by the National Water Resources Council, albeit by infralegal act, based on legislative delegation

inscribed in art. 4, inc. VI of Law 9.984/2000. We believe this legislative delegation to be unconstitutional.

---

[329] Art. 44: It is the responsibility of the Water Agencies, within the scope of their area of activity: XI - to propose to the respective Hydrographic Basin Committee or Committees: b) the amounts to be charged for the use of water resources;

[330] Art. 38: It is the responsibility of the River Basin Committees, within the scope of their area of activity: VI - to establish the mechanisms for charging for the use of water resources and to suggest the amounts to be charged;

[331] TORRES, Ricardo Lobo. Tratado de direito constitutional financeiro e tributario - os direitos humanos e a tributação: imunidades e isonomia. ..., p. 468.

[332] TORRES, Heleno Taveira. Da relagao ..., p. 120 - Footnote 24.

The National Council sets the rate, respecting the volumes abstracted, emitted or released, with a value for each use and each basin. By way of illustration, for the basins of the Piracicaba, Capivari and Jundiai rivers, the rate was set in Annex II of Resolution 52 of November 28, 2005 of the National Water Resources Council.

This Resolution established that, in the basin in question, the basic unit price designated by the National Council would be R$ 0.01 per cubic meter of water abstracted; for the consumption of raw water, it would be R$ 0.02 per cubic meter abstracted for consumption; for the release of organic load BOD5.20 R$ 0.10 per kilogram released; for the transposition of the basin R$ 0.015 per cubic meter abstracted.

In fact, we interpret the combination of all the constitutional provisions as follows.

Law 9.433/97 is not unconstitutional if it fails to set the levy rate in the same law. In fact, the doctrine itself clarifies that the various aspects of the hypothesis of incidence do not necessarily have to be in the same legal diploma, they are often "sparse in the law, or in several laws, many of which are implicit in the legal system"[333] . What we see in the hypothesis of the incidence of water charges is only a justified incompleteness.

In fact, Law 9.433/97 provides for popular participation, through the Basin Committees, in the **legislative process** that will set the rate to be applied. This is where the principle of participatory management (or popular participation) and that of information referred to elsewhere in this work come into play.

Therefore, **the rate must be set by law,** which must be produced with respect for the principle of popular participation. The rate set by an infralegal instrument, such as a Resolution, is an unconstitutional act, as it violates the principle of tax legality.

---

[333] ATALIBA, Geraldo. Hypothesis ..., p. 76.

7.5.5. Personal criteria.

The personal circle will determine the active subject of the tax exaggeration and the passive subject. This element doesn't pose any major difficulties, not least because when we discussed the fully binding activity we showed how the active subject would be. The Union is responsible for creating the exaction, and the taxing power has been handed over to the ANA in the case of "federal" water bodies and to the states, which can delegate it to the Water Agencies, in the case of "state" water bodies.

The taxpayer is the user of water resources in their raw, untreated form. It should only be clarified that water companies throughout the country are, for the purposes of this law, users, as they collect raw water and subject it to sanitary treatment.

Conclusion.

The effort made in this work was to point out viable ways of preserving water resources, in view of the crisis that is only worsening day by day on the national and international scene. The law is an indispensable instrument in the search for rational use of water, since the demand for water only tends to grow - especially in the face of exponential demographic growth, in parallel with human needs dependent on this resource - while the amount of drinkable water in the world is in sharp decline.

We therefore advocate the use of environmental taxation as an instrument to protect water resources. This is because the tax, with all its coercive power, tends to determine the reduction of negative externalities generated by economic activity. Numerous arguments can be invoked in favor of using taxation as a way of bringing regularity to human conduct that predates on water resources. Among them are the economic theories of Arthur Pigou (Pigouvian taxes), Pareto's optimum theory (to control the deficiencies of such taxation) and the theory of fundamental rights.

These arguments are reinforced by an ethical approach, which requires deep reflection on the predatory and irrational system of exploitation of limited and exhaustible environmental resources. Human beings need to stop acting like eighteenth-century owners of the environment (property was an intangible asset and no interference was made in the exercise of this right) and start recognizing the innate value of the biotic and abiotic elements of the "Earth ecosystem".

The intention is not to make a paradigmatic shift in the foundation of law (anthropocentric), even if we were to adopt a biocentric or ecocentric paradigm 157

It wouldn't be easy to overcome the paradox that a system of values, formulated by humans, is justified and only exists because of humans themselves. In reality, what is needed is an awakening of humans to broaden anthropocentrism in order to make environmental protection possible and to recognize the warning cry of the environment.

Recognizing that environmental taxation is a viable path also involves the theory of fundamental rights, insofar as limitations on fundamental rights must be introduced into the legal order through laws.

Environmental taxation is a viable path for the Brazilian legislator to follow. This path was chosen for the preservation of water resources, with the introduction of an economic intervention contribution which aims to ensure that the negative externalities of production are absorbed by economic activity through this contribution, which also has the salutary function of raising funds for the promotion of hydro-environmental public policies.

But the virtues of taxation are not without their difficulties. At this point, it is worth warning of the pitfalls that can be encountered in recognizing taxation as an economic intervention contribution. These mishaps include political and social facts. Taxation is viewed with suspicion by society, especially in Brazil, where the tax burden is heavy and the return in public services offered by the state is deficient. Taxation is also seen as a means of domination and maintaining the power of the rulers, and it is no wonder that it is recognized that there is no power without taxation and taxation without power.

Another serious problem to be tackled is that the contribution for intervention in the economic domain, despite its noble function of preserving the environment, can be diverted to solely finance the structure of the National System. For, not infrequently, the creation of specific funds linked to administrative bodies justifies the contingency of budgetary funds intended to maintain the structure. And even if there is a link between the revenue collected from the tax and the aim of preserving water resources, as there is with social security contributions, there is no guarantee that the revenue collected will actually be applied to the river basin, despite the ingenious accounting provided for in Law 9.984/2000.

Furthermore, the creation of taxes for a preservationist purpose can only be a legitimizing speech to mask the real motivation, which is to supply the public coffers with financial resources to sustain the often corrupted structures of government.

The reallocation of budgetary resources is also common practice, despite numerous constitutional restrictions, a fact that prevents the constitutionally pursued goal from being achieved, in the name, as a rule, of economic stability and the formation of a budget surplus.

Environmental taxation is a discourse that legitimizes the imposition of taxes in order to pursue a noble goal, which is the protection of environmental resources. However, it should be noted that it is not possible to admit, with the environmental crisis we are experiencing, that the imposition of taxes is just a discourse and not a reality.

Another difficulty is the institutionalized and legitimized practice of environmental doctrine, which for a long time held that water charges were a public charge, demanded without the rigors of the tax system. This is also due to a shortage of professionals with interdisciplinary and transdisciplinary training. In fact, the field of environmental tax law is extremely recent and requires interdisciplinary training on the part of the legal practitioner, since the emergence of this new discipline is due to the transfer of methods from the discipline of tax law to environmental law, or vice versa, since the discipline of environmental law itself is already transdisciplinary.

If the collection of water didn't have the rigors of the tax system, respect for the principles of legality and anteriority and the system of immunity of the minimum subsistence level, among others, institutional resistance would be evident, because it's true that taxation generates more security for society than the establishment of public services through the market system. However, the institution that collects these resources is constitutionally bound, making it clear that this is both the way forward and the way back.

Finally, the determination of the tax nature of the Water Law charge has strong arguments to support it, in our opinion more favorable than unfavorable. This is very noticeable because, among other arguments already exhaustively covered in this paper, leaving an increasingly scarce environmental asset under the management of private entities is a risk for society as a whole. As a result, only those who have the economic means to pay for it will have the fundamental right to access water resources that are qualitatively and quantitatively sufficient for survival, a fact that will exclude a significant portion of society from access to this right.

Bibliographical references.

ALEXY, Robert. **Theory of Legal Argumentation: the theory of rational discourse as a theory of legal reasoning**. Translation by Zilda Hutchinson Schild Silva; technical revision of the translation and introduction to the Brazilian edition by Claudia Toledo. 2. ed., Sao Paulo: Landy Editora, 2005.

. **Teoria de los derechos fundamentales**. Madrid: Center for Constitutional Studies, 2002.

ALMEIDA, Caroline Correa de. **Historical evolution of the legal protection of water in Brazil**. Jus Navigandi, Tersina, a. 7, n. 60, nov. 2002. Available at: http://jus2.uol.com.br/doutrina/texto.asp?id=3421. Accessed on: March 3, 2006.

AMARO, Luciano. **Brazilian tax law**. 9. ed., Sao Paulo: Saraiva, 2003.

ANTUNES, Paulo de Bessa. **Environmental Law**. Editora Lumen Juris: Rio de Janeiro, 2006.

ATALIBA, Geraldo. **Hipotese de incidencia tributaria**. 6. ed., 3. tir., Sao Paulo: Malheiros, 2 002.

BARROSO, Luis Roberto. **O Direito constitucional e a efetividade de suas normas** - limites e possiblidade da Constituigao brasileira. 7. ed., Rio de Janeiro: Renovar, 2003.

BENJAMIN, Antonio Herman V. The theatrical state and the implementation of environmental law. *In:* **7th International Congress of Environmental Law - "Law, Water and Life"**, 7, 2003, Sao Paulo.

BOFF, Leonardo. **Ecology: cry of the earth, cry of the poor**. Rio de Janeiro: Sextante, 2004.

. **From the iceberg to Noe's ark: the birth of a planetary ethic**. Rio de Janeiro: Garramond, 2002.

BRAZIL. **National Water Agency - ANA**. Brasilia: Federal Senate, 2001.

BRAZIL. **United Nations Conference on Environment and Development**. 3. ed., Brasilia: Senado Federal, Subsecretaria de Edigoes Tdenicas, 2001.

CAMPOS, Nilson. Water management: new visions and paradigms. *In:* **Water management**: principles and practices. Nilson Campos and Ticiana Studart (Orgs.). 2. ed., Porto Alegre: ABRH,
2 003.

CAMPOS, Nilson; STUDART, Ticiana. Charging for water use. *In:* **Water management**: principles and practices. Nilson Campos e Ticiana Studart (Orgs.). 2. ed., Porto Alegre: ABRH, 2003.

CAPONERA, Dante A. **Principles of water law and administration**: **national and international**. Rotterdam: Balkema, 1992.

CARRAZA, Roque Antonio. **Course in constitutional tax law**. 22. ed. Sao Paulo: Malheiros Editores, 2006.

CARVALHO, Edson Ferreira de. **Environment & human rights**. Curitiba: Jurua, 2005.

CARVALHO, Paulo de Barros. **Course in tax law**. 14. ed. rev. and updated, Sao Paulo: Saraiva, 2002.

. **Direito tributario**: fundamentos juridicos da incidencia. 2.ed. rev., Sao Paulo: Saraiva, 1999.

. **Teoria da norma tributaria**. Sao Paulo: Max Limonad, 1998.

CAUBET, Christian G. **Freshwater in international relations**. Barueri: Manole, 2006.

COELHO, Sacha Calmon Navarro. **Course in Brazilian tax law**. Rio de Janeiro: Forense, 2001.

CUNHA, Luis Veiga da. Half a century of perceptions about water in international politics. *In:* SOROMENHO-MARQUES, Viriato. **The Challenge of Water in the 21st Century: Between Conflict and Cooperation**. Lisbon: Noticia Editorial: 2003.

DANTAS, Fabiana Santos. Water resource management: a critical analysis of Law 9.433/97. *In:* **The application of environmental law in the federal state**. Andreas J. Krell (org.) Rio de Janeiro: Editora Lumens Juris, 2005.

DERANI, Cristiane. **Economic environmental law**. Sao Paulo: Max Limonad, 1997.

DI PIETRO, Maria Sylvia Zanella. **Administrative law**. 16. ed., Sao Paulo: Atlas, 2003.

Private use of public property by private individuals. Sao Paulo: Editora Revista dos Tribunais, 1983.

SPAIN. **Water Law**. Madrid: Ministry of Public Works and Urban Planning, 1990.

FARIAS, Paulo Jose Leite. **Water: economic or ecological legal asset?** Brasilia: Brasilia Juridica, 2005.

FELDMANN, Fabio. Constitutional review and water resources. *In:* MILLAR, Agustin A. (editor). **Water resources management and the water market**. Brasilia: Secretariat of Irrigation, 1994.

FIORILLO, Celso Antonio Pacheco; and RODRIGUES, Marcelo Abelha. **Manual of environmental law and applicable legislation**. 2. ed. Sao Paulo: Max Limonad, 1999.

FIORILO, Celso Antonio Pacheco. **Course in Brazilian environmental law**. 4. ed., Sao Paulo: Saraiva, 2003.

FREITAS, Vladimir Passos de. **Administrative law and the environment**. 3ª ed., 2ª tir., Curitiba: Jurua, 2002.

GERALDES, Andre Gustavo de Almeida. **Legal protection of water sources**. Sao Paulo: Editora Juarez de Oliveira, 2004.

GRAFF, Ana Claudia Bento. State protection over water. *In:* **Waters - legal and environmental aspects**. Vladimir Passos de Freitas (Org.), Curitiba: Jurua, 2001.

GRANZIERA, Maria Luiza Machado. **Water law: legal discipline of fresh waters**. Sao Paulo: Atlas, 2001.

GRECO, Marco Aurelio. Contributions for intervention in the economic domain - parameters for their creation. *In: Contribution for intervention in* **the economic domain and related figures**. Coordinator Marco Aurelio Greco. Sao Paulo Dialdtica, 2001.

GRUPENMACHER, Betina Treiger. Fiscal justice and existential minimum. *In:* **Principios de direito financeiro e tributario - estudos em homenagem ao Professor Ricardo Lobo Torres**. Adilson Rodrigues Pires and Heleno Taveira Torres (organizers), Rio de Janeiro:

Renovar, 2006.

GUERRA, Sidney. **International environmental law.** Rio de Janeiro: Maria Augusta Delgado, 2006.

HARDIN, Garret. **The Tragedy of the Common Good.** Translated by Prof. Tabajara Lucas de Almeida. Available at: http://www.dmat.furg.br/~taba/tragcomum.htm , Accessed on August 1, 2005.

HENDERSON, David R. Biography of Ronald H. Coase. *In:* **The Concise encyclopedia of economics.** Available at: http://www.econlib.org/library/Enc/bios/Coase.html, retrieved on October 15, 2005.

. Biography of Arthur Cecil Pigou (1877 - 1959). *In:* **The Concise encyclopedia of economics.** Available at: http://www.econlib.org/library/Enc/bios/Pigou.html, captured on October 15, 2005.

JUSTEN FILHO, Margal. **The law of independent regulatory agencies.** Sao Paulo: Dialdtica, 2002.

KRELL, Andreas J. **Basic instruments for the management and protection of water resources in Germany.** *In:* Revista Brasileira de Direito Ambiental, ano 2, v. 5, p. 41-72, Sao Paulo: Fiuza, jan./mar., 2006.

. **Administrative discretion and environmental protection**: the control of undetermined legal concepts and the competence of environmental bodies: a comparative study. Porto Alegre: Livraria do Advogado, 2004.

. **Direitos sociais e controle judicial no Brasil e na Alemanha**: os (des)caminhos de um **direito** constitucional "comparado". Porto Alegre: Sergio Antonio Fabris Editor, 2002.

LEITE, 1o8ë Rubens Morato. **Dano ambiental: do individual ao coletivo, exptrapatrimonial.** 2. ed. rev., atual. e ampl., Sao Paulo: Editora Revista dos Tribunals, 2 003.

LUNO, Antonio E. Perez. **Fundamental rights.** Madrid: Tecnos, 2004.

MACHADO, Hugo de Brito. Public Services and Taxation. *In:* TORRES, Heleno Taveira (coord.). **Servigos publicos e direito tributario.** Sao Paulo: Quartier Latin, 2005.

. **Curso de direito tributario**. 24. ed., rev., atual. e ampl., Sao Paulo: Malheiros, 2 004.

. **The concept of tribute in Brazilian law**. Rio de Janeiro: Forense, 1987.

MACHADO, Paulo Affonso Leme. **Water resources - Brazilian and international law**. Sao Paulo: Malheiros Ediotres, 2002.

MARTINS, Ives Gandra da Silva. **A theory of taxation**. Sao Paulo: Quartier Latin, 2005.

MASTRANGELO, Claudio. **Regulatory agencies and popular participation**. Porto Alegre: Livraria do Advogado Ed., 2005.

MEIRELES, Hely Lopes. **Brazilian administrative law**. 14. ed., Sao Paulo: Malheiros Editores, 1989.

MELO, Celso Antonio Bandeira de. **Course in administrative law**. 13. ed., rev., ampl. e atual., Sao Paulo: Malheiros Ediotres, 2001.

MILARE, Edis. **Environmental law: doctrine, case law, glossary**. 3. ed. rev., atual. e ampl., Sao Paulo: Editora Revista dos Tribunais, 2004.

MIRANDA, Pontes de. **Comentarios a Constituigao de 1967**. Sao Paulo: Editora Revista dos Tribunais, 1967, t. IV.

MODE, Fernando Magalhaes. **Environmental taxation, the role of taxation in protecting the environment**. Curitiba: Jurua, 2003.

MOLINA, Pedro Manuel Herrera and VASCO, Domingo Carbajo. Conceptual, constitutional and community framework for environmental taxation. *In:* **Direito tributario ambiental**. org. Heleno Taveira Torres. Sao Paulo: Malheiros, 2005.

MOREIRA NETO, Diogo de Figueiredo. **Course in administrative law: introductory part, general part and special part**. Rio de Janeiro: Ed. Forense, 2003.

MUKAI, Toshio. **Systematized environmental law**. Rio de Janeiro: Forense Universitaria, 2 005.

NICOLESCU, Barsarab. **Transdisciplinary university evolution: a condition for sustainable development**. Available at   :http://perso.club-internet.fr/nicol/ciret/bulletin/b12c8por.htm. Accessed on August 1, 2005.

NUNES, Cleucio Santos. **Tax law and the environment**. Sao Paulo: Dialdtica, 2005.

NUNES, Lydia Neves Bastos Telles. **Property rights and water**. *In:* The protection of water and some implications for fundamental rights. Luiz Alberto David Araujo (Coord.), Bauru: ITE, 2002.

OLIVEIRA, Flavia de Paiva Medeiros de; GUIMARAES, Flavio Romero. **Law, the environment and citizenship**: an interdisciplinary approach. Sao Paulo: Madras, 2004.

OLIVEIRA, Jose Marcos Domingues. **Tax law and the environment: proportionality, open typicity, revenue allocation**. Rio de Janeiro: Renovar, 1999.

STO, Francois. **Nature on the fringes of the law - ecology at the mercy of the law**. Translated by Joana Chaves. Lisbon: Instituto Piaget, 1995.

PAULSEN, Leandro. **Tax Law: Constitution and Tax Code in the light of doctrine and case law**. 7. ed. rev. atual. Porto Alegre: Livraria do Advogado: ESMAFE, 2005.

PIMENTA, Paulo Roberto Lyrio. **Contributions of intervention in the economic domain**. Sao Paulo: Dialdtica, 2002.

. **Constitutional profile of economic domain intervention contributions**. *In:* Contribution of intervention in the economic domain and related figures. Coordinator Marco Aurelio Greco. Sao Paulo Dialdtica, 2001.

PIVA, Rui Carvalho. **Environmental good**. Sao Paulo: Max Limonad, 2000.

POMPEU, Cid Tomanix. **Water law in Brazil**. Sao Paulo: Editora Revista dos Tribunais, 2006.

. **Water resources in the 1988 Constitution**. *In:* Revista de Direito Administrativo, n.186, Rio de Janeiro: Renovar, Oct/Dec/1991.

RIBAS, Lidia Maria Lcpes Rodrigues. Environmental defense: use of tax instruments. ". *In:* **Direito tributario ambiental**. Heleno Taveira Torres (Org.). Sao Paulo: Malheiros, 2005.

RODRIGUES, Silvio. **Civil law**. 23ª ed., Sao Paulo: Saraiva, 1996, v. 5.

SCAFF, Fernando Facury. Reserve of the possible, existential minimum and human rights. *In:* **Principios de direito financeiro e tributario - estudos em homenagem ao Professor Ricardo Lobo Torres**. Adilson Rodrigues Pires and Heleno Taveira Torres (organizers), Rio de Janeiro: Renovar, 2006.

SAMPAIO, Clarissa. **Legality and regulation**. Belo Horizonte: Forum, 2005.

SANTOS, Maria Luiza Wernek dos. The application of the resources obtained from charging for the use of water. The illegitimacy of its limitation. The normative competence of the CNRH and the ANA. *In:* **Administrative Law - Studies in honor of Diogo de Figueiredo Moreira Neto**. Coord. Fabio Medina Osorio and Marcos Juruena Villela Souto, Rio de Janeiro: Lumen Juris, 2006.

SEBASTIAO, Simone Martins. **Environmental taxation**. Curitiba: Jurua, 2006.

SERRES, Michel. **The natural contract**. Paris: Flamarion, 1992.

SILVA, 1o8ë Afonso da. **Constitutional environmental law**. 4. ed. Sao Paulo: Malheiros Editores, 2002.

SILVA, Robson da. **Biocentric paradigm: from private patrimony to environmental patrimony**. Rio de Janeiro: Renovar, 2002.

SOARES, Sebastiao Roberto. **Environmental management and planning**. Available at: http://www.ens.ufsc.br/~soares/aulaG2.pdf. Accessed on: July 9, 2005.

SOUZA, Luciana Cordeiro. **Waters and their protection**. Curitiba: Jurua, 2004.

TABOADA, Carlos Palao. El principio "quien contamina paga" y el principio de capacidad economica. *In:* **Direito tributario ambiental**. Heleno Taveira Torres (Org.), Sao Paulo: Malheiros, 2005.

TORRES, Heleno Taveira. The relationship between constitutional tax and environmental competences - the limits of so-called "environmental taxes". *In:* **Direito tributario ambiental**. Heleno Taveira Torres (Org.), Sao Paulo: Malheiros, 2005.

TORRES, Ricardo Lobo. The taxation of public services in the State of the risk society. *In:*

Public services and tax law. TORRES, Heleno Taveira (coordination). Sao Paulo: Quartier Latin, 2005-A.

. **Treatise on constitutional financial and tax law - human rights and taxation: immunities and isonomy**. 3. ed. Revised and updated up to December 31, 2003, the date of publication of Constitutional Amendment No. 42 of December 19, 2003. Rio de Janeiro: Renovar, 2005-B.

. **The existential minimum and fundamental rights**. *In:* Revista de Direito Administrativo, n. 177: 29-49, Sao Paulo: FGVEditora, jul./set., 1989.

UNESCO. **Great rivers: from conflict to sharing. Infographics: a growing scarcity**. *In:* O Correio Unesco, n° 12, year 29, Rio de Janeiro: FGV Editora, December, 2001.

STATE UNIVERSITY OF CAMPINAS (UNICAMP). **Hydrographic basins: new management of water resources** . Available at : http://www.eco.unicamp.br/ecoeco/artigos/encontros/downloads/mesa3/3.pdf#search='bacias %20hidrogr%C3%A1ficas%20nova%20gest%C3%A3o%20de%20reursos%20h%C3%ADd ricos. Accessed on: July 2, 2005.

VARELLA, Marcelo Dias. **International economic environmental law**. Belo Horizonte: Del Rey, 2004.

VENOSA, Silvio de Salvo. **Civil law: rights in rem**. 2. ed., Sao Paulo: Atlas, 2002.

VERLI, Fabiano. **Fees and public charges**. Sao Paulo: Ed. Revista dos Tribunais, 2005.

VIEGAS, Eduardo Coral. **Legal view of water**. Porto Alegre: Livraria do Advogado, 2005.

YOSHIDA, Consuelo Yatsuda Moromizato. The effectiveness and environmental efficiency of economic, economic-financial and tax instruments. Emphasis on prevention. The economic use of environmental goods and its implications. *In:* **Environmental tax law**. Heleno Taveira Torres (Org.). Sao Paulo: Malheiros, 2005.

ZUMBROICH, Thomas. The European Union's Basic Water Directive as a Result of Changing Awareness in the Protection of Water Resources. *In:* **Local Agenda 21 - participatory management of water resources**. Angela Kuster, Klaus Hermanns (eds.), Fortaleza: Konrad Adenauer Foundation, 2006.

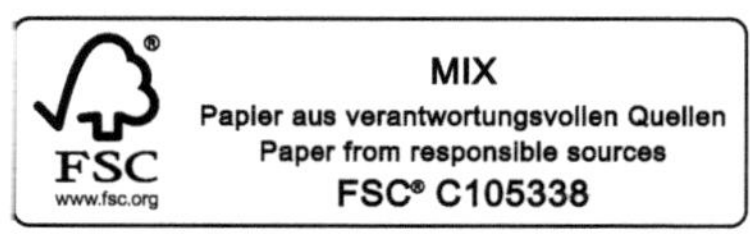

Printed by Books on Demand GmbH, Norderstedt / Germany